MICHIGAN'S HOLY WATER
The Great Lakes Wine Bible

By Rick Sigsby

DREAMBUILDER PUBLICATIONS
Coleman, Michigan

MICHIGAN'S HOLY WATER
The Great Lakes Wine Bible

Copyright © 2013 by Rick Sigsby

All rights reserved. No part of this book may be reproduced or transmitted in any form or by any means without written permission from the author.

Printed in USA by McNaughton & Gunn, Inc.

Copy Editor: Ann Sigsby

Cover photo: Fenn Valley Vineyard by Bob Gudas

ISBN: 978-0-615-87437-1

PREFACE

Thomas Jefferson said, "Good wine is a necessity of life." And truly, the best way to learn about wine is to drink it. Despite being literally ignored by the wine world, Michigan wineries have much to be proud of and the time is right to drink up and start the bragging.

In the last decade, while in the midst of a depressed economy, the Great Lakes wine industry has shown unprecedented growth and the number of acres dedicated to grapes have increased dramatically. Michigan is producing award-winning wines – not first place in the local wine club tasting contests but rather prestigious events across North America and internationally.

Historically, Michigan has been producing great wine "legally" since the mid-1800s and shortly after Prohibition ended, the state was a national leader in the wine industry – for heaven's sake, Cold Duck was invented right here in Michigan! Yet, the rest of the country has failed to take notice. Strohs was brewed in Michigan but it was Martin Luther who said, "Beer was made by men, wine by God."

Thus, the idea for a book touting great tasting Michigan wines was born.

A quick literary search showed the last quality book on Michigan wineries (*From the Vine*) was published in 2007. Statistics from the Michigan Wine and Grape Industry Council show the number of wineries in our state has more than doubled since 2006, from 45 to 93 in 2012. When looking at regional and national writings about wine, Michigan is barely a footnote.

The Wines of America (1990) dedicates five pages of a 530-page book to the Michigan wine industry. *The Modern Encyclopedia of Wine* (1991) has three paragraphs about Michigan in a 576-page book. *The Great Wines of America* (2005) mentions one Michigan winemaker. *The Wine Bible* (2001) doesn't mention Michigan at all. To add a touch of insult, neither does *Wine for Dummies* or *The Idiots Guide to Wine*.

It is time Michigan had its own wine bible – Martin Luther may have been a bit bold in his statement but a multitude of palates would agree that Michigan has an abundance of blessed winemakers. In the Great Lakes state, from the Upper Peninsula to the Indiana/Ohio border, from the Lake Michigan shoreline to the Huron waters, Michigan wineries are making holy water in the form of great wine.

This book has an insider's look at why every resident should have their wine racks filled with Michigan wine and every tourist should never pass a wine tasting room without stopping. From $5 to $50 bottle, the price is right because the wine in Michigan tasted heavenly.

Table of Contents

Introduction..6

Acknowledgements..8

History of Michigan Wines..9

Myths & Mysteries..14

Michigan Wineries..20
    Northwest
        Old Mission..................................20
        Leelanau....................................... 46
        Other..118
    Northeast..151
    Southwest...176
    Southeast..272
    Yooper Wine...325

From Vine to Dine..336
    Have Wine – Will Write............................337
    Three Tier Distribution System..................343
    Starting a Vineyard....................................347
    Distributors..351
    Retailers...357

Wine Clubs...376

Bibliography/Photo Credits......................................380

About The Author..381

Directory of Wineries...382

Sponsors...390

Introduction

Dear Wine Enthusiasts,

The Michigan wine industry has a rich and colorful history. It is one part nature, two parts determination with a little charm thrown in, to make it a celebration of life with great tasting wines.

My grandfather saw the potential for making quality wine here back in 1936, when he moved his Meconi Wine Company from Detroit to Paw Paw and it became the St. Julian Winery – the oldest and largest winery in Michigan. My father advanced the industry further by creating the first tasting room at our winery with the opening of I-94 in 1959. Today, tasting rooms are a permanent feature at virtually every winery in the state.

The first major wine producing area was actually in the downriver area of southeast Michigan but it soon moved to the western side, which now has the largest American Viticultural Area – the Lake Michigan Shore AVA - with over thirty wineries in primarily Berrien, Cass and Van Buren counties. Traverse City's wine country began with pioneers like Bernie Rink (Boskydel Winery) on the Leelanau peninsula and Ed O'Keefe (Chateau Grand Traverse) on Old Mission peninsula. Now northwest Michigan has nearly fifty wineries.

There are over one hundred wineries sprinkled all over the state including the Upper Peninsula and weekend warriors hit the wine trails the year-round. Even as the vineyards go to sleep for the winter, wine lovers flood the tasting rooms in search of Michigan's latest great vintage.

But it's not just the wine they seek...it's the story behind the winery that also intrigues them.

Every vineyard and every winemaker has a story. It's a family owned farm with generations of experience or a young couple getting their hands dirty with a plot of land that now sprouts grapevines. It's an entrepreneur who has gone from making wine in the basement to scratching off another item from their "bucket list" by starting a winery.

Michigan has reason to brag about its wines. We have something for everyone – red, white, dry or sweet. The industry was built on the backs of Concord and Niagara grapes but now boasts world-class vinifera and fruit wines that will please the palates of nearly every wine drinker.

What better way to enjoy this book, than to get a bottle of Michigan wine and learn about our fascinating industry. Believe me when I say we have plenty of "chartacters" to talk about. Sip some of our "holy water" as you turn the pages, going from winery to winery around our state. It's a journey you will savor.

David Braganini, St. Julian Winery

Acknowledgements

The origins of this book started with a conversation at the Bay City Wine Club – "why aren't more Michigan wines represented each month?" When no one came up with an adequate answer, my friend Phil said, "Rick, that sounds like the subject of your next book."

This book could not have been written without the cooperation of the dedicated vineyard managers, winemakers and winery owners of the Michigan wine industry. There was no intent to slight any that didn't get interviewed but a big thank you to the ones who did. Special kudos to Marie Chantal Dalese of Chateau Chantal and Lee Lutes of Black Star Farms for being great sounding boards and to David Braganini of St. Julian for writing the introduction.

Sommelier Tom Fischer and Karel Bush of the Michigan Grape and Wine Industry Council were instrumental in assisting with industry contacts. As with several previous books, this project wouldn't have been possible without the assistance of Phil Paulus, Tom Noxious and my wife/editor Ann.

Disclaimer

No doubt, there are errors in this book. By mutual agreement between the author and editor, they were left intentionally. As there are people whose purpose in life is to seek out all literary abnormalities, it was a vain attempt to appease all our readers.

THE HISTORY OF WINE

First Came the Grape
Then Came The Wine

In the beginning, God created grapes. Shortly after, man created wine.

The word "wine" and its various synonyms appear in the Bible over 200 times. Its first reference is in the book of Genesis. Noah's ark floats around for over a year and upon debarkation on Mt. Ararat, he becomes a farmer. And what does he plant?

Genesis 9:20 – "Noah, a man of the soil, began the planting of vineyards."

Then after harvesting the grapes...

Genesis 9:21 – "He drank of the wine and became drunk..." Thus, Noah became the first vintner and wine drinker. And in his defense, he had no concept of a hangover. Also, for those that dismiss the health benefits, Noah lived another 350 years after drinking the wine and died at the ripe old age of 950 years old.

The history of wine is as elusive as the hints of essence in a fine Riesling or Cabernet. Every ancient civilization drank and worshipped wine in some form or another. Archaeologists have found evidence of grape wine dating back to 7,000 BC in Georgia, a former part of the U.S.S.R. (not the more familiar state of the original thirteen colonies). The earliest remnants of a winery date to 4,100 BC in Armenia.

The Greeks not only drank wine but they created Dionysus, the god of wine and revelry (a great combination). The Romans adopted this god and changed his name to Bacchus.

In medieval Europe, wine became the social drink of all the classes. Some of the largest producers were the Benedictine monks, who had vineyards in Bordeaux, Burgundy and Champagne – Dom Perignon was a Benedictine monk.

Leif Erikson carried wine on his Viking vessel to seek new lands to the west. Ironically, one of the first things he and his men discovered upon landing on North American shores was a large cluster of wild grapes. Erikson promptly declared this vast wilderness Vinland, which translated to Wineland for the non-Scandinavians. They immediately started making a vintage for the journey home.

Christopher Columbus also brought several European grape varieties to the New World. He stocked his three ships with barrels of wine and rationed it primarily to counteract the crew almost constantly whining – 'how much further?' and 'are we there yet?'

Other Old World grape varieties were brought in from the south by the Spanish conquistadors and Spanish missionaries were the first to establish a wine industry on the west coast.

MICHIGAN'S WINE HISTORY

The history of wine in Michigan also began with early explorers who found an abundance of wild grapes and fruit along the rivers and streams. A French missionary named Jacques Marquette established the first permanent settlement (1668) and it's assumed that wine was an important part of everyday life – he's a Frenchman after all. Antoine Cadillac established the first documented vineyard at Fort Pontchartrain (present day Detroit) in 1701.

As the French began expanding to the suburbs of the Fort, they discovered the downriver region to be laden with grapevines and called the nearby river *La Riviere au Raisin* or the Grape River- which is known today as the River Raisin in Monroe County. This undoubtedly prompted the establishment of the state's first commercial wineries. It was also the site of a major battle during the War of 1812 between British and American forces from which came one of the great rallying cries "Remember the Raisin." (I'm not making this up!)

In 1868, just thirty years after Michigan became the 24th state, Joseph Sterling opened the Pointe Aux Peaux Wine Company in Monroe. That same year, A.B. Jones started a vineyard in Paw Paw, which has remained a cornerstone in the wine industry ever since.

By the 1880s, Monroe had over 1000 acres of grapevines. But within a few decades, grape rot and the temperance movement would doom the vineyards in the southeast Michigan area and the downriver area never recovered.

However, by then several wineries had opened in southwest Michigan. An American physician named Thomas Welch recognized the grape growing potential of the region. He opened a Welch's Grape Juice facility in Lawton (four miles from Paw Paw) in 1919 just prior to the 18th Amendment ushering in the Prohibition Era.

Mariano Meconi moved his winemaking operation from Windsor to Detroit after Prohibition ended in 1933. He relocated to Paw Paw in 1936. One of the Meconi Wine Company's most successful labels was a sweet Concord wine called St. Julian, named in honor of his Italian hometown patron Saint San Guiliano. Shortly after Pearl Harbor was bombed, the company name was permanently changed to the St. Julian Wine Company, which grew to become Michigan's largest winery.

From 1933 to 1984, one of Michigan's significant wine producers was the Bronte Champagne and Wines Company in Detroit. Their primary contribution to the history of wine was the introduction of Cold Duck to the market in 1964, which quickly became their best seller. In fact, its success caught the attention of Ernest Gallo in California and prompted him to create the Andre' brand, which is still on the retail shelves today.

Vineyards in northern Michigan got a toehold when a librarian named Bernie Rink began experimenting with French-American hybrid grapevines on the Leelanau peninsula in 1964. He opened the Boskedyl Winery tasting room in 1976. By then, fellow entrepreneur Ed O'Keefe had planted a vineyard on the Old Mission peninsula in 1974 and opened the first commercial wine operation in the north called Chateau Grand Traverse.

The Leelanau AVA (American Viticultural Area) was established in 1982 and the Old Mission AVA came along in 1987. Now the Traverse City area has over 30 wineries with labeled wines for sale.

In 1981, the Fennville AVA was the first in the state and only the 3rd in the U.S., with Fenn Valley Vineyards its only commercial winery. The Lake Michigan Shore AVA covers over a million acres of southwest Michigan and has over two dozen wineries in Berrien, Cass and Van Buren counties.

Now other wineries are springing up in various non-traditional fruit growing areas of the state. Southeast Michigan is making a comeback; the eastern or 'sunrise side' along Lake Huron is thriving and even the Upper Peninsula boasts several wineries and tasting rooms.

There are now over 120 licensed wineries in Michigan and 101 of them are members of the Michigan Grape and Wine Council, which means at least 51% of their wine is produced from Michigan grown fruits. The history of Michigan's wine industry is certainly colorful and definitely has a bright future.

THE MYTHS AND MYSTERIES OF WINE

Let your wine age – it will taste better.

Instead of looking at wine like scotch or whiskey, think of it as fresh fruit. Most wines are not meant to age. If you're buying wine in a store, it's already aged on the shelf. If you're buying it from a winery, ask them about the longevity of the wine. The value rarely goes up by storing it in your basement for years.

Red wines go with meat – white wines go with fish.

There are no hard and fast rules. Read the labels, consult the experts (take their advice), experiment, stick with what you like.

Looking at the color of wine will tell you how it tastes.

They tell you to look at the edge of the wine in the glass, for indicators as to the age of the wine and how it might taste. If it's cloudy it might not taste good…dah, ya think?!
If it's clear, it's a young wine, if it's yellowish or brown tinted, it may have some age – pure wine swill! The way to determine the taste is to TASTE the wine.

Look for the 'tears of wine' or 'wine legs' - that will indicate more alcohol and a better wine.

No, it just means you'll get drunk faster. The alcohol level doesn't equate to quality.

Each style of wine needs its own style of glassware.

This is a myth created by glassware companies. Pick a glass you like to go with reds and pick one that goes with whites. Save on cupboard space and dishwater hands.

Open your wine a few hours before drinking to 'let it breathe.'

This is a good idea if your wine as developed a bad odor but that also indicates a more deep-seated problem. The difference in taste if you don't let it breathe isn't worth the time sitting around waiting. Go out and splurge on a $10 wine aerator or if you think it's better to spend $40 on one, go for it…or do like me, which is spend the money on a good wine and let it breathe in the glass.

Old wine eventually turns to vinegar.

If wine is stored properly it can still taste great after many years or *vino caveat emptor* (wine buyer beware). Even if a connoisseur stores it, a wine can just become old, uneventful or bland. As with people, some wines don't age well. The death knell for wine is being exposed to air – cork dries, cork shrinks, air rushes in, wine goes bad. It could turn to vinegar but more likely it just goes sour and DON'T cook with it.

Sniff the cork.

Poser! Just look to see if the cork is wet or moist. If so, there is a 99 out of 100 chance the wine is fine. After a few sips, you'll know if the wine is bad. Then go back and check the cork. An expert MIGHT tell by sniffing – leave it to them. Sniffing is a rookie play. Hint: a cork should smell like…cork.

Holding a glass by the stem and swirling your wine is snobbish.

Rule of thumb or in this case hand: Reds taste better at room temperature and whites should be chilled. Cupping the glass – body heat – you get the idea. For most people, swirling your wine is a mimicking habit but not a bad one. Maybe you're just contemplating or pondering a thought. Actually, the swirling does release aromas that should enhance the drinking experience. Just don't spill the reds on white tablecloths – the hostess will get pissed.

Every party store or winery has a wine expert.

Do you really think the kid stocking the shelves at Wal-Mart knows a good wine to go with your fabulous rib roast tonight? Most wineries do a great job of educating their tasting room staff, but not all. Most party stores don't have an expert but each town usually has a 'go to guy' (examples: Gar Winslow in Midland or Matt Rhodes in Okemos) – ask around, it's worth it to know who these people are.

After opening a bottle, you need to drink it all because wine starts going bad immediately.

This is a tricky one because of the drinking and driving laws. Finish the bottle because you want to, not because you feel you have to – if you're eating and drinking with friends, the second bottle could get you in trouble driving home. Finish'em both off if you're not going anywhere. Some wines actually taste better the next day. Don't throw it out because you think it will taste bad later.

Twist or screw off caps are just for cheap wines.

This goes back to the days of Boone's Farm but let's hope you've graduated and moved on. Actually, some really high-end and even smaller 'boutique' wineries are using the twist or screw caps for closures. It eliminates the storage and cork taint issues and makes it much easier to re-close the bottle for 'I think I'll have some more wine later' (see above). Many wineries would jump on the bandwagon but it's also a more expensive type of closure.

You're getting a higher quality wine if it says Reserve or Estate on the label.

It could mean you're getting the wineries' very best or it could mean this bottle was the last of 100,000 cases sold overseas from last year's vintage. There is no industry consensus for the usage of the word 'reserve' and 'estate' could be the neighbor's backyard. It actually refers to the fruit being grown on land owned or controlled by the winery. Both terms *can* mean this is a very special wine – again, ask the experts first.

Dom Perignon invented champagne and said 'come quickly, I am drinking the stars.'

The earliest recordings of 'sparkling wine' were about 100 years before our famous monk was born (circa 1531). There is evidence that he had something to do with perfecting the mushroom cork and wire closure for champagne but the quote came from a 19th century ad campaign, about 200 years AFTER Dom was gone. There is no doubt that some of the very best champagne in the world carries his name.

The first United States commercial winery was in California.

Wrong. This is a hugely debated issue but only amongst old wineries. Obviously, the first winemakers in North American were the Scandinavians – they named their discovery Vinland after all. There were winemakers in Florida around 1563; Virginia in the early 1600's and Pennsylvania by the mid-1600's – of course, these weren't states yet, just areas on old crude maps. Indiana claims the title for the first commercial winery in 1806. Missouri also claims the title. Ohio claims to be the home of the first 'successful' winery. Californian monks were making wine in the 1700's but it was supposedly so bad they couldn't sell it to anyone. Michigan's first commercial winery was in Monroe in 1868.

European wines are better tasting than American wines.

Rent the movie *Bottle Shock*. It tells the true story about a blind wine tasting contest in France back in 1976. French judges placed an American red and an American white wine #1 – it shocked the wine world and of course, the French immediately tried to dismiss the results.

In Michigan, the wine experts usually come from MSU.

This is a tough call (cuz I'm a U of M grad). But the acknowledged expertise in growing fruit actually does come from Michigan State University. They have an excellent viticultural program. Lee Lutes, winemaker for Black Star Farms, hates the term 'expert' when it comes to wine but he did graduate from MSU – in FINANCE! Larry Mawby, one of the most knowledgeable people in sparkling wines, did graduate from MSU – in ENGLISH! Dr. Charles Edson, an MSU professor – in HORTICULTURE...okay, I give up.

All wine lovers are snobs.

See low, guttural tongue flapping Bronx cheer, ppthhfffftp...shame on you for thinking that.

Michigan Wineries

Northwest
Old Mission..20
Leelanau...46
Other..118
Northeast...113
Southwest..176
Southeast..272
Yooper Wine.......................................325

Northwest Old Mission

Brys Estate...21
Chateau Chantal......................................27
Chateau Grand Traverse..........................33
Hawthorne Vineyards..............................39
Peninsula Cellars....................................41

BRŶS ESTATE VINEYARDS AND WINERY
The Accent Is On Elegance

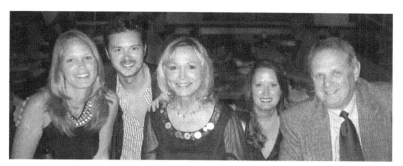

Brys – Katie, Patrick, Eileen, Stephanie, and Walter Brys

Sometimes when a seed is planted it lays dormant for many years before sprouting. Such is the case with Walter and Eileen Brys. Shortly after marriage, a trip to Napa Valley in the mid 70's fostered a dream that would eventually become Brys Estate Vineyards and Winery on Old Mission peninsula.

Walter excelled in real estate development, which eventually took him and his family to Texas. His son Patrick, who serves as Brys Estate operations manager, said, "Our family always joked about my father building 'destination resorts' and in Texan translation that means he built prisons (laughing)."

While Patrick was in California getting a degree in marketing, Walter and Eileen retired and moved to Florida while still in their 50's. Life was good – for a few months until they became 'bored to tears.' Then that memorable trip to Napa, which had become a 'bucket list' dream to start a winery, reemerged. They began a two-year search of the wine regions of the United States for the right place and in 1999 chose an 80-acre former cherry orchard on Old Mission.

After hiring a vineyard consultant, the land was refurbished, vines were planted and the renovation of the 1890's farmhouse began. The farm transformation was amazing and for their efforts the Brys' were recipients of the Peninsula Township Development Award in 2003.

Cornel Olivier also came on board that year as winemaker to oversee the development of the vineyard and the new state-of-the-art winemaking facility, which was completed as the first crop of grapes were being harvested in 2004. Another South African winemaker, Coenraad Stassen, came over from Chateau Chantal to join the Brys team in 2007 as Cornel left to begin developing 2 Lads Winery a little further up the peninsula.

As the winery continued to grow, Walter and Eileen began looking for more second-generation involvement. Patrick had spent summer vacations from his job in L.A. helping in the vineyard and was eventually called home to take over the day-to-day operations. "In 2009, I actually thought I'd try it for three months," Patrick said. "That quickly became nine months, so I bought a home here in 2010. The winery has doubled in size since then so my job description has changed but there's still only 24 hours in a day (laughing)."

The winery originally produced award-wining Riesling and dessert wines but now has committed fifty percent of their 40 acres of grapevines to produce red wine – with good reason. Their 2011 Merlot won Best of Class in the heart of prime competition – California! Brys Estate is becoming known as the 'go to' place for great red wines. Oh, and their whites are still winning awards as well.

Interview with Patrick Brys:

What were the determining factors that led your parents back to Michigan and the land that became Brys Estate?

Patrick: They really did their homework. They revisited Napa Valley, Oregon, New York and actually considered several other properties in the Traverse City area. This land had all the right things – soil composition, slope, micro-climate, etc. Plus, we have family here and it reminded them of when they first visited Napa Valley – back when it was still mostly family owned wineries and wasn't so commercialized. They saw quality in an emerging wine region.

It is hard to believe the before and after pictures of the old farmhouse.

Patrick: Yes, my mother says she was looking at that rundown homestead through rose-colored glasses – we said it looked haunted (laughing). Rather than rent a home on the water during the remodeling, my dad bought a 'land yacht', i.e. a mobile home, and they lived on the property until the new home was completed. They had never owned a 'used' house before but they also really felt a historical connection to the entire property.

With two South African winemakers, is there a major difference in your winemaking process from other wineries?

Patrick: Each winemaker has personal differences. Both Cornel and Coenraad brought South African winemaking influences to Brys Estate, but to answer the question – major differences, no. I also think its fair to say I'm a bit prejudiced in thinking the subtle differences makes our wines a little better.

How does the family feel about having their name on the label?

Patrick: My mother sent lists around to all the family and all her friends – vote on your top three choices. She'd refine the list and send it out again. In the end, my parents wanted the winery to be a family business. I have two sisters who have periodically helped and my cousin is the tasting room manager. We are proud of what my parents built here and we all take pride in having our name on the labels.

Your title is Operations Manager. What does that entail?

Patrick: I tell everyone I basically do everything no one else wants to do. With the increase in size and sales, my job has gotten more complicated in the last four years but I love it. I look at the big picture – the overall wine production, month-end reports, marketing, media relations...but I also make sure I'm scheduled to work several days in the tasting room – especially Saturdays. When you have a thousand customers come through here, it really puts my organizational skills to the test (laughing).

How do you think the public perceives Brys Estate?

Patrick: I think it's somewhat looked at as a hidden treasure. We're on Blue Water Rd., a little ways off Center Rd, which runs the length of the peninsula. Many times we've heard customers brag about 'discovering' Brys Estate. We are a boutique size family-owned winery and people like the quaint but elegant looking facility. We're been producing 100% estate grown wine for three years now – so we are building a reputation for having more discerning but affordable wines that aren't being mass produced.

Your slogan seems to address that – Taste The Estate Difference.

Patrick: Yes, a grower is in the business to sell grapes by the ton. Our winemaker actually starts making the wine well in advance of the harvest through the selection process. We cut back and leave a lot of fruit on the ground – so only the very best grapes go into the wine. Less fruit brings out the intensity and concentrated flavors.

One of your award-winning wines is Dry Ice, a dessert wine. Explain ice wine.

Patrick: We leave the fruit on the vine until the plant shuts down for winter. The grape begins to dehydrate and concentrate the flavors. When the temperature drops below 15 degrees for two consecutive days, we know the water in the grapes is completely frozen. They are picked and sent to the press immediately – sometimes you get only a few drops of nectar per grape. We say each sip is like drinking a whole cluster. A normal size bottle of wine has 600 to 800 grapes – a ½ bottle of ice wine could have over 2,000 grapes in it. That's why dessert wines are so expensive but it's REALLY good – like liquid gold.

Describe your parents using wine adjectives – then yourself.

Patrick: My dad is jovial, easy going and a relaxed guy – I would say he's like our Pinot Noir/Riesling blend. It's easy to drink, not too formal and something that goes with a great conversation. My mother is into the details. She's a Pinot Noir – something that requires attention and detail, when treated right it turns into an amazing product. And me – I'd like to think I've taken the best of each parent – so I'm a nice Rosé (laughing).

After a scenic trip through the vineyards, the tasting room destination is the reward – thanks Patrick.

See the Brys Estate ad on page 396.

CHATEAU CHANTAL
Wine With a Touch of Divine

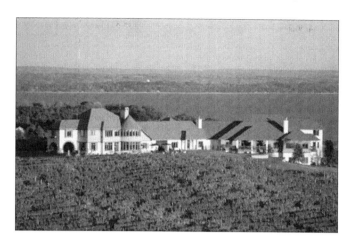

Could it be possible for a winery to be inspired from sacramental wine? Indeed, it could.

In the case of Chateau Chantal, it's certainly possible considering the founders are a former priest and nun. Most wineries have an interesting background in regards to their origins but this is a wine tale of un-orthodox proportions.

Listeners usually stare with raised eyebrow when a tale starts with 'I know this is hard to believe but this one IS true.' Chateau Chantal's origins began in the Sacred Heart Seminary and convent of the Felician Sisters of Detroit. "It does make a great tale," said Marie Chantal Dalese, daughter of Robert and Nadine Begin, founders of the winery. "They had great careers in Catholic service, which made them fantastic hosts for what they do today and what they started on this hilltop on Old Mission Peninsula in 1993."

Robert was ordained in 1960 and served as a priest in various parishes throughout Detroit until 1972, when he made the decision to start his own construction company. Nadine entered the convent in 1950 and served the Catholic Church for 22 years before 'getting a fresh taste of life outside the walls.'

"My parents knew each other and worked together but there's no crazy Thornbirds chapter," laughed Marie. "For different reasons and at different times, they ended their church careers." Whether it was fate or divine intervention, their paths crossed again, a romance was kindled and they married in 1974.

So where did the inspiration to start a winery come from? "I've never discovered my father's original thoughts that inspired Chateau Chantal," Marie said. "But he does admit learning a lot about wine from his Monsignor, who happened to be from Bordeaux."

Marie came along in 1978 when her mother was 46 years old and her father took his entrepreneurial spirit to Old Mission Peninsula in 1980. His vision of building a European style winery chateau became clear while cross-country skiing on 'the hill' that also happened to be for sale. The Gore cherry farm became the Begin Orchards in 1983 and the planting of vines began in 1986.

Special permits were obtained from the Peninsula Township because no one had ever attempted a multi-purpose operation – a winery, a tasting room, a bed & breakfast, and private residence, all in one building. After its completion in 1993, the 3-room B & B started taking reservations, the Chateau served up their first vintage with Mark Johnson coming on as winemaker and the Begin family moved in – Marie was fifteen years old.

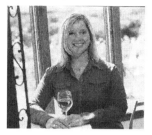

Interview with Marie-Chantal Begin Dalese:

There are investors and a Board of Directors but were your parents the ones who named the winery?

Marie: Yes and obviously there were a lot of discussions and decisions about the business around the house prior to moving into the chateau. It was Chateau Chantal this and Chateau Chantal that and Chateau Chantal shut up (laughing). At the time, I wasn't interested in wine at all, so it was tough on a teenager girl for a while. And my father was very emphatic about me trying the product. I was twenty-one before I could sample the family wines! (laughing)

How did your labels evolve?

Marie: The original label was a more European styled look – you know, with the picture of the chateau on display. Our reserve labels still have that look, although the building has changed over the years with several expansions. The non-reserve wines feature smaller detailed pictures of this place.

Two of your original wines are Naughty Red and Nice White. Are there religious overtones in those names?

Marie (chuckling): No, actually Mark was flipping through a magazine and saw a wine described as 'being so naughty it can be paired with fish.' In fact, many of our customers were told of the health benefits of red wine but liked the taste of whites. So Mark developed a low tannin, non-oak barreled red wine with a smooth taste to satisfy those people. The Nice wine is a bit sweeter and both are still some of our top sellers.

So eventually that teenager girl grew up and started working for her namesake. Tell us about that journey.

Marie: My dad always asked me to work elsewhere, so I worked in restaurants and retail stores throughout high school and college in Chicago – eventually getting a degree in Marketing/Management from DePaul University. There was talk about maybe someday coming back to Chantal but no serious discussions. I was always encouraged to follow my own path. A seminar on wine marketing resulted in me taking a graduate wine marketing program in Australia for a year. I made friends there who came from around the world, the program was fantastic and I met my husband Paul there – we met at a wine tasting. I came back to the States and worked for a few years at a wine retailer and then for a distributor, got married and moved back to Traverse City in 2009. I had no interest in being 'the daughter who works in the family business.' But my degree at DePaul was tailored to the wine business and my advanced studies in Australia lend credibility to my work here.

And now, your husband Paul works here as well...

Marie: He's a diesel mechanic by trade and now is our viticulturalist. Wine making can be labor intensive but there's a lot of machinery involved as well and so he's fixing things all the time – and I can't tell you how handy that is to have a mechanic on staff!

Have you seen any tasting room trends over the years?

Marie: I think initially the customers gravitated toward sweeter wines but surprisingly our top five wines are very diverse – from a sweet late harvest Riesling to our Malbec, which is a dry red, with Naughty and Nice and a bubbly called Celebrate in there. The major shift we've seen here is lower wine by the bottle sales and an increase in wine by the glass, with the change in the law allowing us to charge for a 'tasting.' There is no quantity measurement placed on what a 'tasting' is but our customers have really taken to a glass of wine with some food. Of course, with our view up here, it's a great setting for that as well.

What is your current percentage of sales from the tasting room?

Marie: We've gone from virtually all our sales being out of the tasting room in the early years to about 50/50 with statewide retail distributors. But the profit margin drops significantly with each set of hands that touch the bottle before it gets to the consumer.

Yes, that is true in the book business as well. Your parent's story would make a great book.

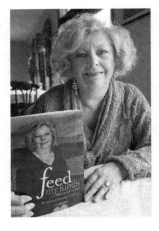

Marie: Well, now that you mention it, we did delve into the publishing business when my mother wrote about her journey and put it with her favorite recipes. And she is a shameless promoter (laughing). She has a captive audience at breakfast with guests staying at the B&B. She's such a charmer and puts the bite on everyone of them – 'did you know the recipe for what you're eating this morning is in my book?' At eighty years old, you get a hug, a story and an invite to buy her book (laughing).

Ask her if she'd add this book to her pitch? Much thanks Marie.

See the Chateau Chantal ad on page 399.

CHATEAU GRAND TRAVERSE
O'Keefe's Folly Becomes The Mothership
Of Northern Wineries

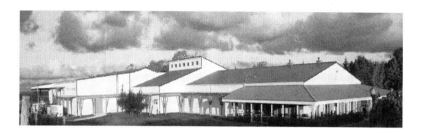

With a 55-acre parcel on Old Mission Peninsula, Ed O'Keefe started planting European vinifera grapes in 1974. They became the first commercial winemaking operation in northern Michigan. In the beginning, it was known as O'Keefe's folly but now, nearly 40 years later, Chateau Grand Traverse produces over 110,000 cases of wine annually.

"We grow grapes; we make wine; we sell wine – not a very fancy business plan but that's what we do," said Eddie O'Keefe III, second generation President of Chateau Grand Traverse. The operation has expanded to 120 acres of grapes spread out over four vineyards, making eighteen wine varieties under three different labels.

For an Irish kid from Philadelphia, starting a winery in Michigan makes a fabulous story to begin with. The highlights include being a world-class gymnast; serving in the Airborne Special Services; becoming an undercover criminal investigator with the Treasury Dept.; and building/operating nursing homes – all these before O'Keefe's love of wine, which he acquired while serving in the army, brought him to Old Mission Peninsula.

While researching the area around his summer home near Traverse City and consulting with a multitude of grape growing experts, O'Keefe became convinced that European vinifera grapes could grow in northern Michigan. The path was far from smooth, but with the help of his two sons, Eddie and Sean, Chateau Grand Traverse has become a world class wine making facility from the highpoint of the peninsula, with a spectacular view and great selection of award-winning wines.

Interview with Eddie O'Keefe:

To say the least, your father took a unique path to get into the wine business...

Eddie: Yes, my father is a colorful man. He is Irish Catholic and my mother is a Wisconsin Norwegian Protestant and right after they were married, they moved to Miami to work in the Jewish Community Center – obviously, a marriage made in heaven (laughing). When he sold the nursing home business, he took the capital gains and put it into a "loss carry forward" business, which is a large cash upfront enterprise where you expect to lose money for an extended period – that's how many of the California wineries started in the late '60's and early 70's. My dad chose Michigan.

So in 1974, it all began as O'Keefe's folly?

Eddie: Many of the locals made reference to the quote 'a fool and his money are soon parted.' My dad told them all (in a more colorful manner) to take a flying leap. We've never wavered from our mission, and we've put almost everything right back into the business.

When CGT started in the 1970's the cherry was king and now grapes dominate the landscape. Why the big turnover?

Eddie: First, land in this desirable scenic area is at a premium price. Second, it takes much more land to grow cherries commercially. Five acres of land on Old Mission Peninsula will produce approx. 20 tons of grapes or 3,000 cases of wine – a small but thriving business. Those same acres with cherry trees don't get your foot in the door.

The past perception and prejudice was 'if it comes from Michigan it can't be a good wine.' How did you overcome that?

Eddie: Our Riesling is one of the best – anywhere. It comes from quality fruit, not quantity. I always called it 'judo marketing.' That is, taking your opponent's momentum or in this case, their perception and flip them – have you tried the wine, then let'em taste it, tell the story and gradually, one by one they become loyal customers.

What is the history behind the Chateau Grand Traverse name?

Eddie: It started as the Grand Traverse Vineyards and then changed to Chateau Grand Travers – the French spelling. But so many people kept asking 'what happened to the e?' So, we finally just added it – why fight it (laughing)? Sean and I always said the Chateau moniker kept our foot in the '70's. Anything with Chateau attached to it was very chic back then.

And now you have three brand names. How did that come about?

Eddie: We produce the wines we like, what we need to make and what the customer wants. Most wineries develop secondary wine names – they go to different markets and have different price points. Our Chateau Grand Traverse labels are premium grapes grown on site. Grand Traverse Select wines are a blend of sourced juice and the Traverse Bay label is primarily for our cherry wines. Those two secondary brands are our 'survivor' or 'insurance policy' brands when our vineyard production suffers from bad weather, which happened in back-to-back winters in 1994 & '95. We were first criticized for doing that but when it happened again in 2003, many wineries began to understand our strategy.

What percentage of your wines is Michigan grown?

Eddie: The CGT and Traverse Bay are 100% Michigan. For the Select label we primarily use a Washington grower who we've worked with for over 20 years and who grows grapes to our specifications for the Select label. Interestingly, we are one of the largest retail wine sellers out of the tasting room but one of the lowest by percentage in overall sales.

How does the pricing work and how did you expand into regional markets?

Eddie: My dad and Sean's careers are much more interesting – I'm the boring one in the business (laughing). Long story short, I learned the distribution/pricing part from driving a truck and working with distributors. The distributors and retailers have a basic set mark up, so from our end, we have to price each label accordingly to get a $9.99 or $14.99 bottle of wine on the shelf. Things like pallet pricing and 'just in time' inventory or next day delivery all helped. Starting with a quality product and proper pricing have built up our brand name and resulted in the expansion from 5,000 cases when I started in 1985 to where we are today.

It's turned out to be a pretty good living...

Eddie: Yeah, if you just could eliminate the hard work (laughing). Perception is everything. People see us flying off to Europe – yes, it's nice but we're not spending time in Paris. We're out in wine country working. People like to think of owning a winery as an 'easy road with a silver spoon' existence, when in reality, wineries are just glorified farms.

Wine isn't a necessity – it's a luxury. How do you explain the rapid growth in Michigan during a down economy?

Eddie: In my opinion, there are several reasons. After 9/11, we all said 'oh @#$%, what now?' Initially, everything came to a standstill but eventually, local and in-state people started saying 'let's not go to California, let's go up north', which perpetuated 'let's support and buy local.' It's interesting you said wine is a luxury. About a year ago, I went to a conference where Nielsen research did a study on things that went away because of this latest depressed economic. They looked at wine in the grocery stores and determined the market basket had changed – wine purchases remained steady so it officially moved from luxury item to a necessity. Basically, the shopper was saying 'I'll cut back on some items but I'm not giving up my wine.' That's why wine is still a growing business – great wines at great prices.

Okay, finally – pick a wine that best describes you, Sean and your father.

Eddie: I'm the Dry Riesling – straight forward, goes with anything; Sean is Gruener Veltliner – up & coming, unique and interesting; and my dad is a rich, robust, full-bodied Late Harvest Riesling with a lot of character!

Three Aces, thanks Eddie.

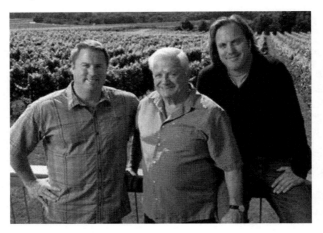

Chateau Grand Traverse – Eddie, Ed, Sean O'Keefe

See the Chateau Grand Traverse ad on page 400.

HAWTHORNE VINEYARDS
From wine what sudden friendship springs!

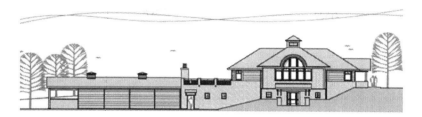

Hawthorne Vineyards is the 8th winery on Old Mission Peninsula to open a tasting room. Bruce and Cathleen Hawthorne had the Grand Opening in May 2013 but they jump-started the operation by opening the cellar for guests in 2012 while construction of the winery was happening all around. It's never too early to promote good wine.

If you're looking for a secluded scenic view of both bays without traffic noise and an eloquent, personable setting, Hawthorne's is the place. If you start to get the feeling of being in the only vineyard around, you are in tune because it really IS the only winery off Peninsula Drive overlooking the West Bay, and is only four miles from Traverse City. Take the short winding road (Camino Maria) through the woods to the top of the ridge and you emerge into Hawthorne's world of wines.

Both Bruce and Cathleen have family roots in northern Michigan and get back to home turf as often as possible. Bruce is a corporate attorney for a large defense contractor and Cathleen, already a Master Gardener, is currently enrolled in the University of California Davis winemaking program Their love of wine became apparent when they purchased the 80-acre site from Chateau Chantal in 2005.

Chateau Chantal was using a few acres for source wine and there was already a small cherry and plum orchard on the property. The Hawthorne's immediately planted an additional 26 acres of vines and have plans to expand again in the future.

Brian Hosmer, a protégé of Chantal's Mark Johnson, is the winemaker and has produced four 2010 wines for the tasting room – a Cabernet Franc/Merlot blend, a reserve Chardonnay, a reserve Pinot Noir and 26 cases of Lemberger, which has already sold out!

Cathleen's fingerprints are all over the winery design. With a desire to make the facility friendly and intimate, major features include a private tasting room, an outdoor wine patio with fireplace and a spectacular view. Meant to be a seasonal operation (May thru October), the fireplace does offer an opportunity to enjoy a glass of wine on weekends later in the year.

Although Hawthorne Vineyards is a joint operation with Chateau Chantel, the new winery will be offering entirely different wines and incorporating innovative farming techniques. Currently, 80 to 90% of their wines come from their own property with the remainder of the fruit made up from the Old Mission Peninsula area.

It may be secluded but the Hawthorne's are making it worth the trip.

See the Hawthorne Vineyards ad on page 407.

TIME TO GO TO SCHOOL
WITH PENINSULA CELLARS

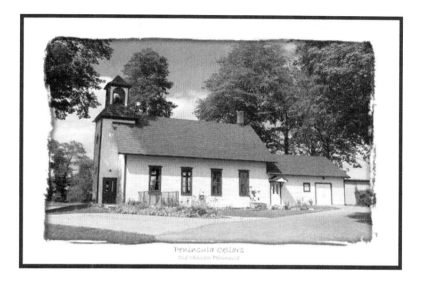

The Old Mission peninsula saw Dave and Joan Kroupa open winery #4 in 1994. Although their grapes were young, their fruit and family roots date back to the earliest days of farming in the area.

"Our son John represents the sixth generation Kroupa farming up here," said mother Joan. "Dave's great grandparents grew some of the first cherries on Old Mission peninsula. More fruit trees were added – apples, plums and pears - each generation expanded the property. Now we have nearly 300 acres and 30 acres of grapevines have been added starting in 1991."

Lee Lutes came on as their first winemaker in 1994. He utilized Dave's skills as a master handyman and started cranking out batches of great wine from plastic tanks. "It was a good match –

we were just getting started and Lee was eager to ply his new trade," said Joan. The business quickly expanded and the word went out for additional help. Another native son, Bryan Ulbrich, came calling. When Lutes left for Black Star Farms in 1998, Bryan assumed the winemaking duties. That year the Kroupas also moved their tasting room into the 1896 one-room schoolhouse on M-37, which runs the length of the peninsula.

When Ulbrich left to start the Left Foot Charley winery in 2007, John Kroupa became the Headmaster of the winery operation. Under his leadership, Peninsula Cellars has continued to thrive. And based on the number of cars parked at the schoolhouse, there are a lot of students enjoying the wine.

Interview with Joan Kroupa:

The Kroupas are truly one of the taproot families on the peninsula. How has the landscape changed over the years?

Joan: The peninsula has always been agriculturally based but the residential areas are growing all the time. The township has done a good job continuing to promote agriculture and managing the land instead of allowing the area to be overrun with housing. The cherry business has always been up and down so we were lucky to get into the wine business when we did. I don't know what the ceiling is on growth but I've heard many times, people don't want to see Old Mission turn into another Napa Valley with there being one winery after another.

Who planted the seed to put grapes on the Kroupa property?

Joan: Our neighbor, who had a vineyard, encouraged Dave to plant some vines and pretty soon that evolved into starting a winery with them. After about eight months and realizing we had differing opinions on the direction of the business, we bought them out. I guess that's how it's been on almost everything we've done – we jump with both feet and are all in (laughing). We've been very fortunate to keep moving forward going from Lee to Bryan to John as winemakers.

How did you decide on the name Peninsula Cellars?

Joan: We were so eager to get started and we came up with a bunch of names. It was 'fits and starts' to begin with…mostly false starts (laughing). Our farm has a beautiful view and we just love this area. We kept coming back to that theme and eventually Peninsula Cellars was the simplest and easiest way to express it.

And I see you've incorporated an old map of the Old Mission peninsula on your logo and wine labels.

Joan: Yes and we did learn a few things along the way. Before someone started copying our creation we trademarked the logo. Our reserve wines feature the location map and winery name. The other wines feature our schoolhouse tasting room location and both are working very well.

That just means you're doing a great job getting customers to identify wines with your location. Who came up with the clever schoolhouse names?

Joan: The family and staff have roundtable discussions. We came up with names everyone can relate to, like Detention and

Homework. The Old Schoolhouse Red & Whites were just a natural – by consensus, everyone agreed they fit. You can imagine how many names we've come up with that have a schoolhouse theme. We'll never make that many wines (laughing).

I would assume most of your grapes come from your vineyard but do you use 100% Michigan fruit?

Joan: Almost all of it comes from our vineyard and Old Mission peninsula. We also contract with a grower in Frankfort, Michigan who has a great Pinot Noir supply.

Tell us about the *Time* magazine article that gave your Select Riesling an 'excellent' rating.

Joan: It was a total and pleasant surprise to us – we didn't even know the article was coming out. The author selected one wine from each of the 50 States and rated them from Excellent to Good, Bad or Undrinkable. I think our wines can compete with anyone but it's nice to get recognition from an 'outsider.' He didn't just pick his favorites, because I think there were nearly as many wines he rated undrinkable as he deemed excellent. (Actually, Joel Stein rated 12 State wines excellent and only six undrinkable but he also rated 13 other wines as bad)

Most farmers get satisfaction from growing something from the land, but is there a difference between growing cherries and grapes?

Joan: I can't speak for others but it is different for us. With our cherries, the satisfaction ends when they are sent to be processed because we don't know where they end up and what the end product will be. But with our grapes, we have more control and see the end results and the satisfaction comes from the customer enjoying our wine. With the winery and tasting room, we get to share the whole experience with others through our wines. They ask us about the process from the grape to the bottle of wine and we are able to tell that story.

Now you're also expanding the Peninsula Cellars tasting experience to southeast Michigan. Tell us about that.

Joan: Yes, a young couple named Cortney and Shannon Casey have opened a tasting room in Shelby Township called Michigan By The Bottle. They picked six Michigan wineries to showcase their wines – Peninsula Cellars being one of them. I think it's a wonderful opportunity to reach a different market.

And it's another opportunity to hear your story and try your wines. Thanks Joan.

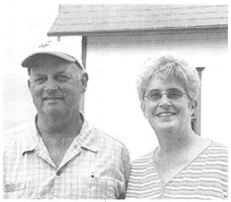

Dave and Joan Kroupa, Peninsula Cellars proprietors

NORTHWEST LEELANAU

BEL LAGO..47
BigLITTLE..54
BLACK STAR...58
BLUSTONE..63
BRENGMAN BROTHERS................................70
CHATEAU de LEELANAU.................................78
45 NORTH 84
GILL'S PIER..89
GOOD HARBOR...95
L MAWBY..101
ONE WORLD WINERY....................................106
WILLOW..112

Wine a bit – You'll feel better.

BEL LAGO
Beautiful View, Beautiful Wine

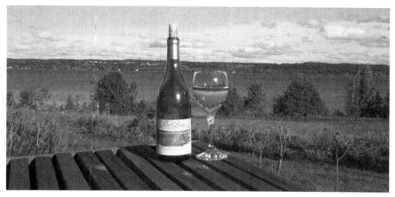

There is no doubt, as you gaze across the vineyards overlooking Lake Leelanau, the owners are stewards of the land and have an appreciation for beautiful things. Dr. Charles (Charlie) Edson and his wife Dr. Amy Iezzoni, both happen to be horticulturists and wine lovers. They, along with Amy's parents Dom and Ruth Iezzoni, are the architects of those vineyards and created Bel Lago Winery just so visitors can enjoy their wines and the view with them.

Charlie went to the University of Michigan for three years before realizing horticulture was his true love, which prompted a transfer to MSU. "I have nixed all school loyalties and it causes me no strife whatsoever," he chuckled. With a Masters degree in apples, Charlie discovered Stan Howell, the Director of MSU's Viticulture program and signed on as a research technician to get his Doctorate.

From there, he went to the University of Missouri for four years, working with the grape and wine industry helping growers improve their production practices. He also met and eventually married Amy, who is now a world-renowned professor at MSU in fruit plant genetics. Charlie also returned to MSU for research and some guest lecturing.

While still in Missouri, he planted a test plot of wine grapes on his father-in-law's property on Leelanau peninsula in 1987. Prior to becoming a vintner himself, Charlie pruned vines for Bruce Simpson of Good Harbor Winery and Larry Mawby of L. Mawby Vineyards. "They became two of my mentors," he said. "They both taught me a lot about the practical aspects of owning a vineyard and winery."

Over the years, they expanded to three estate vineyards, with 30 of the 90 acres in vines, planting over 100 different varieties of wine grapes. One of them is the French white grape called Auxerrois. Bel Lago not only was the first in Michigan to plant it but they were also the first in the nation to get a label for that variety.

The tasting room was opened in 1999 on S. Lake Shore Dr. It's obvious they've put their horticultural background to good use when viewing the environmentally friendly landscape. Even the natural tones of the building make it look like it's coming out of the hillside.

Bel Lago offers a selection of seventeen wines including Auxerrois and their 2011 Jefferson Cup award-winning sparkling wine Brillante NV.

Interview with Charlie Edson:

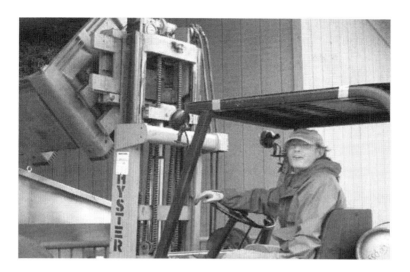

Was there an Aha moment to start the winery after planting the grapes?

Charlie: It was more of an evolution. We started to move forward by planting Pinot Grigio around the winery property in 1992. It was doing well in our test plots and I personally like that wine. Most people associated Pinot Gris and Grigio with Oregon and Alsace, France and I'm a big fan of those two grape growing regions.

Did the name Bel Lago speak to you or were other names considered?

Charlie: My father-in-law Dom's first language was Italian. He was sitting on our hillside one day – thinking in Italian and thinking what a beautiful lake he was looking at. We were all trying to think of a name for the winery. He came down the hill and said 'I've got it – Bel Lago', which is beautiful lake in Italian. Consequently, several of our wines have Italian names – Primavera is Italian for spring and Tempesta is Italian for storm.

You use a variety of interesting labels. How does the choosing process work?

Charlie: Our original label was a commissioned artwork of the vineyard across the road from the winery. A graphic artist developed the Bel Lago script. We keep that on every label and

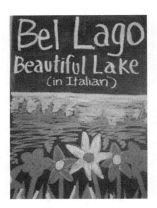

it's always contrasted and distinct enough to read from a distance. Bruce Simpson told me a long time ago that fifty percent of the people will love your labels and the other fifty percent will say 'what were you thinking?' And he was right. Recently, we've been using some of my daughter's drawings and the public really likes them.

Bel Lago has won numerous awards and you've been a judge at numerous competitions. Give us your take on the wine rating system.

Charlie: Judging wine is totally subjective but they do try to frame what a judge should look for to be consistent in their evaluation of each wine. In basic terms, a bronze medal wine should be sound with no flaws. Silver constitutes a wine with special qualities that make it stand out. A gold medal wine stands out as an example of that variety wherever it's grown. For double gold, the wine has to be a unanimous gold awarded at more than one table of judges. Best of Class means you've beaten all the golds in that class – Best of Show means you've beaten all the Best of Class. The rules are a little different at each competition but as the quality of wine improves, the competitions get harder. Today, a gold medal is much more significant at a major competition because the quality all over the world has improved dramatically.

When deciding on what wines to bottle, how does that selection process work?

Charlie: The final decision is mine but I don't rely totally on my palate. Everyone's palate is different so I have a panel of tasters that work for me to help. We also will do trials in the tasting room to get customer opinions on the finalists for certain blends. I take notes on everyone's comments and when we do a final blend I'll bring out a wine from the past to see how the current wine stacks up to a previous vintage.

So it's your choices that ultimately puts your stamp on a Bel Lago wine and makes it different from other winemakers?

Charlie: First and foremost, is the quality of your fruit but after that we all have access to the same basic tools. So it comes down to how you use those tools. You've heard the expression that 'wine is science and art.' I liken it to an artist who has the same palette of colors – each artist chooses how to place those colors on the canvas.

There are over 100 varieties of grapes at your disposal – how many do you use in your winemaking?

Charlie: Actually, we're using almost all of them. Why so many? Here's the thing, blends are very complex – we may use from 15 to 25 different varieties in one blend. It could be 50% Cab Franc and the rest - as many subtle varieties it takes to make it a great tasting wine. It's much like a chef cooking and adding as many spices as it takes to make his specialty. What's interesting about blending is, occasionally, as little as 1% of a variety can materially change a taste and be very meaningful.

Bel Lago was for sale – is it still on the market?

Charlie: It is but we'd only consider selling to the right buyer – someone who would take care of what we've created here. If we don't find that person, we'll keep going on. Winemaking is a very satisfying business. A couple years ago, I was sitting at a restaurant on the Hudson River in New York drinking a glass of our wine that happened to be on their wine list – that was a lot of fun.

Matt Rhodes of Dusty's Cellar in Okemos told me about a food and wine 'taste off' between you and Lee Lutes at Black Star Farms. So who won?

Charlie: (laughing) We were both left on the floor beaten and bloody. Really, those tastings are a lot of fun and everyone comes out a winner. We both take it seriously and are passionate about our wines. When you are dealing with quality wines, it comes down to a question of style. It is a very interesting, educational and entertaining evening for the guests – that's what it's all about.

Tell us about Auxerrois (pronounced awk sehr WAH).

Charlie: It's a white grape I discovered in Alsace, France and introduced it to Michigan. When I tasted it and the more I learned about it, I thought it would really make an impact back home and it has. We're very proud of that. It is a short season variety and we have a short season climate. Therefore, on Leelanau peninsula, when we harvest the grape it still has enough acidity to give it backbone and can be a stand-alone wine. People love it – I just wish more could pronounce it (laughing).

I can pronounce Bel Lago, and I'm glad we had this chat – thanks Charlie.

I'm dreaming of a white Christmas but if the white runs out, I'll drink red.

BIG PLANS FOR GREAT WINES AT bigLITTLE WINERY

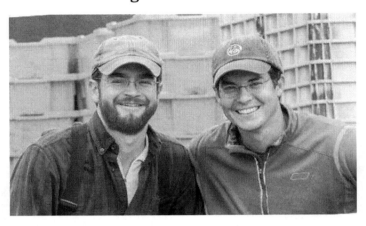

Two brothers, Pete and Mike Laing, started making wines on Leelanau Peninsula in 2010 from grapes grown on their parent's property. Pete has a beard – Mike doesn't; Pete was an engineer – Mike was a teacher; one is big – the other is little. Together, they own the bigLittle Winery and are one of the newest winemaking operations in Michigan.

Under the tutelage of Larry Mawby, owner/winemaker of the L. Mawby and M. Lawrence labels, the brothers are producing a refreshing style of bold wines. It is evident from the names of their wine, which reflect fond memories from their childhood, they want to share those fun times with everyone.

It all started with retirement plans, when their parents bought an old cherry farm on the peninsula in 2001 and dad planted a few acres of grapes to make a little wine. Mike was in Chicago teaching math, while Pete was in Virginia working for a credit card company. It became apparent retirement disappeared when the grapevine plantings expanded to eight acres and the Laings partnered with Larry Mawby.

A love of the land and a strong desire to work together brought the brothers back to Michigan and the genesis of the bigLittle winery was sparked. Being neophytes to winemaking, they fully intended to start small and grow with experience. So it is surprising to see their wines already being distributed throughout Michigan.

"We didn't need a distributor just out of the starting blocks but Cherry Capital Foods was fairly new and was just starting Up North Distributing," said Mike. "We thought it was a good opportunity to grow together. Years down the line, I think we'll look back and thank ourselves for not trying to grow too fast."

However, their wines are off to a fast start.

Interview with Pete and Mike Laing:

So what inspired the name bigLittle Winery?

Mike: We struggled coming up with the right name. The idea just popped into my head one day and wasn't immediately rejected by Pete (laughing). It highlights the bond between the big and little brothers but also is interchangeable on who's coming up big – depending on each other's strengths. Hopefully, the name also fits our style of wines. We are a small winery but intend to produce big-bodied wines.

What are the origins of your clever labels?

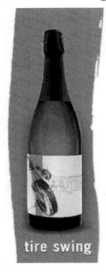

Pete: The names of our wines represent childhood memories – Tire Swing, Crayfish, Treehouse, Mixtape…things we did together growing up in Ann Arbor and up here.

Mike: Much like Larry Mawby has done, we thought it would be best to have the winery and wine names be a reflection of ourselves. It comes out more naturally when talking about the product and us – living the brand, so to speak.

You don't have any formal training as winemakers. What's the most surprising thing you've learned about the whole process?

Pete: I think you'd be surprised at the number of winemakers up here who were never "educated" to be winemakers and just carried on after years of on-the-job training. Larry is obviously our 'go to guy' but we also consult with several other winemakers as well. I'd say the biggest surprise and also a critical factor in maintaining a quality product is cleanliness – 80% of the job is keeping the equipment and winery clean.

How are you trying to separate yourselves from other wineries?

Pete: We are offering a different style of wine on familiar varieties. An example would be making a white Pinot Noir, where most others are making a red Pinot Noir or Larry making a Blanc de Noir with that grape. We are also blending Riesling with several other varieties, which is uncommon up here. The intent is to stay true to our goal of making wines that are the best from this area.

And the next step is a tasting room?

Pete: Yes, it will be a small friendly atmosphere. No pretensions – snobs not welcome (laughing). We're not a Chateau…and we want to make it fun for our customers, much the same as the L. Mawby tasting room.

Where do you see bigLittle in the near future?

Mike: Right now, we are 100% Michigan grapes grown on our parent's property and bottled right here on Leelanau Peninsula. That won't change in the immediate future but as we develop our craft, we may expand and experiment after we've established a quality brand name.

What's the most satisfying part of starting this new winery and the most frustrating part?

Mike: We always wanted to work together, so I'd say the most satisfying part is working with Pete.
Pete: The most frustrating part is working with Mike (laughing).
Mike: I guess I shouldn't have jumped in there so quick!

Ah, brotherly love…it's obvious that you work well together (two brothers – one dream) and that has produced some big wines from a little winery (small batches – big wines). Thanks guys.

DOWN ON THE VINEYARD WITH LEE LUTES AT BLACK STAR FARMS

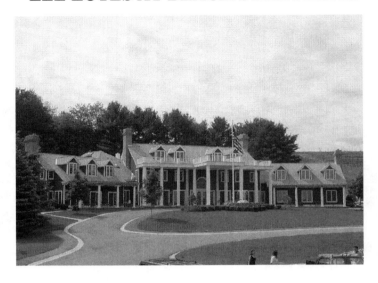

It's an Inn, a riding stable, a farmers market and it's a winery – a very good winery with Head Winemaker (he doesn't like the word Executive) Lee Lutes overseeing the production of award-winning wines on both peninsulas. To look at the main 'farm' on Leelanau, it breathes class but with a country cottage atmosphere. On Old Mission, the Black Star Farms tasting room has the 'come into my house and try my wine' look and Lutes is at home in both places.

He is a native of the Traverse City area but with a lot of European and Australian influence running through his veins. The table at home always included wine. "I remember my parents drinking wine with dinner," Lutes said. "When I was real young, they let me try some but it was usually Cold Duck for me (laughing)."

In the back of his mind were fond memories of a youthful 3-year hiatus in Australia and after obtaining a degree in finance and a brief stint as a stockbroker, the wanderlust drew him back down under. "I rekindled friendships and eventually embarked on what became a wine walkabout," recalled Lee. "It was an adventure into learning the wine business and it really lit a spark in me."

Upon his return to the States, he worked briefly for a New York wine importer and then helped manage the wine list for a Manhattan restaurateur. "I got a great education and learned the ropes in the underbelly of the big city – it was tough on a green Midwest boy…I was eaten alive out there," laughed Lutes.

After returning to Michigan, he began working at Peninsula Cellars in 1994 and took them from a very small operation to selling nearly 5,000 cases annually. Then Black Star Farms came calling. "Ironically, I turned them down twice," Lee said. "It never was 'an offer he can't refuse' but they did say 'what's it gonna take' and they are great partners to work with."

He handles the wine operation and the others work the 'hospitality' side, although the winery includes a lot of hospitality for the growers and customers as well. The original plan was for the winery to eventually become a 10,000 case facility but their success quickly outgrew the Leelanau farm, which warranted expansion to the Old Mission location.

The man is always busy working with his team of people in the winemaking process or educating the tasting room staff, strategizing a new marketing campaign or dealing with distributors, but on rare occasions you can catch glimpses of him.

And despite his youthful looks, that Midwest boy describes himself as being nearly twenty vintages old.

Interview with Lee Lutes:

What makes the Black Star Farms operation unique?

Lee: It truly is an agritourism business, but from the winery portion, we have formed a co-op atmosphere with the growers benefiting downstream from a quality product produced. I honestly think because of the time span and individual talents that have come together, the model we've generated can't be duplicated. Our growers are also shareholders, which has contributed to the consistency and high quality of fruit for our wines...all made from 100% Michigan fruits.

Tell me about the relationship between the growers and the processor or winemaker. Is your relationship different?

Lee: Typically, it's an adversarial relationship, in that the grower is paid by the pound and the winemaker is seeking higher quality fruit, which in this climate means lower yields or less fruit per acre. So you need to strike a balance. We've done away with that formula – our growers are paid the following year based on the retail price of the wine. Therefore, it's in their best interest to produce lower yield/higher quality grapes, which in turn produce a higher quality/higher priced/higher profit wine.

What separates you from other winemakers?

Lee: There is a lot of ego involved with winemakers but the reality is the process at the basic level hasn't changed much in a couple thousand years – its not rocket science. In my opinion, the difference here is we pay attention to the details. I say 'we' because this isn't a one-man operation. It's many people working together, not one person working with many. The details start with the growers and include the other owners who understand and appreciate the necessity of having expensive equipment, quality packaging, a willingness to hire creative talents and be open to creative ideas – with the underlying premise being quality first and foremost. We believe in the concept of 'terroir' (French for earth or soil in relation to place), which means our wines taste like they come from here and we work hard to maintain that quality from vintage to vintage.

You have tried thousands of different wines but have you been able to educate your palate to know what the public will like, even if it's a wine you personally might not prefer?

Lee: That, in the nutshell, is the key to making any winery a success. If you can't make the right decisions on which wines should be bottled, then you end up with a lot of unsold wine. I can think of several wines in our tasting room that I wouldn't reach for to take home for dinner but are some of our biggest sellers. Our success comes from not only producing what we like but also what the consumer wants and where they see value.

Because of your experience 'in the trenches' so to speak, does anything surprise you anymore?

Lee: It still surprises me when I hear someone, who I think is trying to give me a compliment, say 'this is really good wine – I mean REALLY good.' My first thought is 'did you expect mediocrity?' But I also get great satisfaction out of taking people beyond their expectations and I think we do 99 out of 100 times.

Originally, I assume Black Star Farms recruited you for your winemaking abilities but your role here has grown considerably from those beginning years. Beyond just making wine, what do you consider your strongest asset?

Lee: There are quite a few winemakers who make lousy managers but I would say my strongest asset is the ability to wear many hats and wear them reasonably well...most of the time (laughing). I try to be an 'everyday' manager and not micro-manage, which I've been accused of doing in the past. I like to give people responsible jobs and let them do it but I also like to deal with potential problems in real time rather than wait for weekly meetings. It seems to be getting easier the older I get.

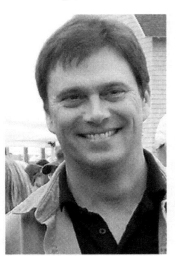

Where do you see yourself between now and when you are, say, forty vintages old?

Lee: I don't ever expect to completely retire. It may sound like a cliché but I truly don't look at this as a job. At some point in the future, they might let me mow the vineyards and I'll still be happy being around the grapes. And of course, I can always make myself available to sip wine with our customers.

Now that doesn't sound much like a job either. Thanks Lee.

BLUSTONE VINEYARDS
Worth The Time To Find

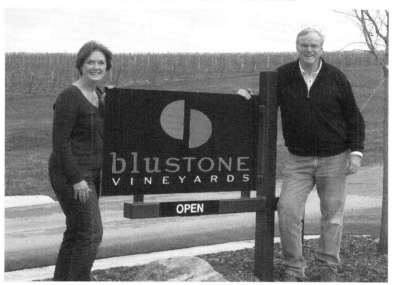

It's a rare, beautiful find...words to describe the elusive Leland Bluestone. Although not that difficult to find, you could easily use the same words to describe Blustone Vineyards on the Leelanau peninsula. You won't find an 'e' in Blu but you will find award-winning wines.

Tom and Joan Knighton started visiting northern Michigan about 25 years ago. They were so captivated by its beauty, that 13 years ago they built a home overlooking Lake Michigan.

Tom is a management consultant working with executives all over the world. "I'm blessed to have a profession that allows me to work out of my house," he said. "All I need is an internet connection and an airport and I'm in business."

One of the pleasures Tom and Joan, a retired teacher, enjoy on their travels is wine and winemaking in various parts of the world. Closer to home, they started getting serious about winemaking on the peninsula about five years ago. "We enjoy wine and were looking for something we could share as a family with our two sons," Tom said.

They began talking with winery owners and winemakers about the direction of the wine industry in Michigan. They were convinced that the industry was vibrant and growing, having personally observed the dramatic increase of wineries near their home. "After doing our homework, we knew it was possible to put the right pieces together to make good wines and also create an experience for customers that would keep them coming back," Tom recalled.

"Our mission is to make wines people respect and to connect people to the beauty and bounty of the land."

Their 40-acre farm was purchased in 2010, with eight acres of five-year old vines already producing great fruit. "Before ever signing on the dotted line, I tried a glass of the owner's private stock and loved it," chuckled Tom. Because the vineyard was already producing, Blustone's first two vintages wines were allowed to gracefully age prior to their release when the tasting room opened in November of 2012.

Don't be surprised to see Tom behind the bar serving you one of their ten wines, putting up another piece of fabulous photography highlighting the surrounding land or working out in the vineyard.

Interview with Tom Knighton:

You were quoted as saying your tasting room 'blurs the lines between the outdoors and indoors.' Could you explain that?

Tom: I said that? Wow, that's exactly what it feels like – that's pretty good. We specifically built the tasting room with a lot of glass to see out over the vineyard because we want people to feel like they are a part of the process of growing grapes and making wine. Seeing people sitting on the patio or out on the grass, literally next to the vines, enjoying our wine – that's the experience we wanted to share.

The vineyard name is Blustone – what happened to the 'e'?

Tom: We got rid of it (laughing). There's nothing special about the word Bluestone, so we dropped the 'e' and it fits with the more contemporary nature of our brand. An interesting thing happened when we had our first MDOT sign installed out on the M 204 highway. I drove by and they'd put an 'e' in there for us. I called the person in charge of sign projects and he said 'I guess someone thought they'd help out these people who can't spell.'

Your name actually comes from the Leland Bluestone – is that correct?

Tom: We wanted something distinctively Leelanau and since our home is on the beach, we love to walk and admire the stones that have washed up on the shore. . Every once in a while, you come across a piece of Leland Bluestone. It's an exciting, unexpected moment because it is a rare find. That's what we want to create with our wines and experience – an unexpected moment of delight - – much like finding a piece of bluestone on the beach.

The bottle labels are certainly distinctive...

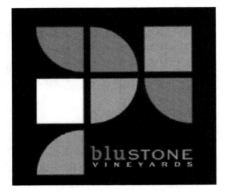

Tom: If you look at, for example, our Chardonnay label – it is a modern representation of the beach rocks. What you see is the grays, whites, blacks and the distinctive bluestones sticking out from the rest. We wanted to create a modern vibe and a contemporary feel in our graphics, our tasting room and our labels. Each label is different but with a contemporary feel to it.

I read a quote from you – 'We let the wine express itself.' Is that your wine philosophy at Blustone?

Tom: We do as little as possible to the wine – we let it do what comes naturally. We learned a lot from our very first wine, which was an unoaked Chardonnay. We met with Shawn Walters, our winemaker, to taste it a few months after the crush. We thought we'd be aging it in oak barrels but Shawn encouraged us to 'listen to the wine – it will tell you what it wants to be.' It was telling us it was beautiful just the way it was and since that day our Chardonnay has remained 'naked' without the influence of oak. That's how we approach all of our wines - we allow the vineyard and the terrior to express itself.

What's the story behind Winemaker's Red and Ad-Lib wine?

Tom: Winemaker's Red is not estate grown but rather a Michigan wine. We look for the best combination of grapes available across the state to make a unique blend every year. It's aged in very interesting barrels with alternating staves of French and American oak, which simultaneously softens the tannins and creates great mouth feel. The 2011 vintage released in 2013 won a gold medal in California, which we're really proud of. Ad-Lib is the wine we make after everything is done (laughing). It was born out of the bounty of the 2011 harvest – we had lots of fruit left over so we put it all together to create a fun wine. Unashamedly, it's our hamburger, spaghetti and pizza wine. Not totally surprising, it's also one of our best sellers.

Congratulations on winning so many awards for such a new winery. Tell us - how much wine do you have to send to those contests and do they send you back a critique of your wines?

Tom: The tasting contests are all different. One contest sends you tasting notes if you win double gold (which means a unanimous gold by the judges), which is really helpful. Mostly, we want to see how our wines measure up to the best in the world. We tend to go to international competitions where there are enough wines entered to get a sense of the industry and market – 2,000 to 3,000 wines from 30 to 40 different countries. You are invited to pay an entry fee and send 3 to 6 bottles of wine. Sometimes the competitions have a big gala afterwards and use the event to raise money for charity, so there's a benefit as well as a critique of the wines.

You mentioned seeking advice from other winery owners. Can you share some of that advice?

Tom: We talked to several winery owners in the area and asked what makes some wineries succeed and others struggle. We were told, like any good business, you need a good plan and have good business disciplines (crossing your fingers doesn't hurt either). Another owner said 'let me be perfectly honest – some people have romantic ideas about owning a winery. The reality is I spend 10% of my time growing grapes, 10% making wine and 80% of my time selling it. If you don't enjoy selling your wine, don't get into the business.' I think we got good advice.

Prior to opening, you held a rather big family event at your tasting room site – your son got married.

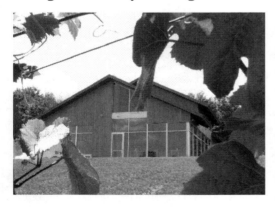

Tom: We thought the tasting room would be done by September, but if you've ever been involved in construction you know delays are almost inevitable. We were hopeful but in hindsight, not all that realistic. I told our contractor we HAD to have power and lights. We put up a big tent and looking back at pictures of the wedding, you can see a 2/3 done tasting room with construction sheeting on the exterior walls. On top of that, because of the hot summer, our crew was already harvesting Pinot Gris. They were driving out as the wedding party was coming in. All in all, it was a fabulous day and evening – we did have lights!

So then you opened a few months later on a Leelanau 'Toast the Season' event weekend. How did that go?

Tom: I took the risk of advertising we'd be open for the event and we were moving things around and bringing in wine the night before. It was kinda crazy but a really successful opening. I was so proud of our team. Something like 800 people showed up. Joan had a dream the night before…remember the ending to the movie Field of Dreams, with all those cars coming up the drive…that's exactly what she saw when we put the open sign out.
It's nice to hear about dreams coming true – thanks Tom.

See the Blustone Vineyards ad on page 395.

Wine (n): A hug in a glass.

JOIN THE FAMILY AND HAVE SOME FUN AT BRENGMAN BROTHERS CRAIN HILL VINEYARDS

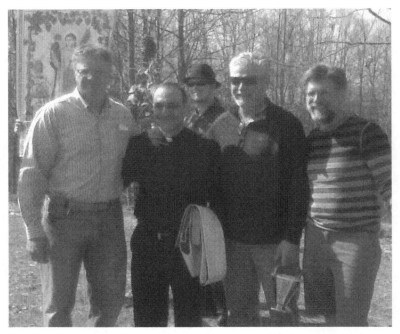

Brengman Bros – Gerald, Father for blessing, Ed, Robert, Nathanial Rose, wineworker (background)

If you need a vision for a Michigan vineyard, look west as you reach the crest of Crain Hill Rd. on Leelanau peninsula. The Brengman Brothers picked this location to start their own vision of creating a premium wine-producing vineyard. At the end of the winding drive is a winery that speaks 'come join the family, escape - relax and enjoy our wine.'

The family patriarch, 'Captain' Brengman was a bricklayer for thirty years before entering the restaurant business in east Detroit. Having built a labor force of thirteen children came in handy (eight boys, five girls). "As the clan grew, we kept moving until we finally settled in a big house that would hold us all," laughed the Captain.

Many of the siblings took up the hospitality mantle at some point in the various Captain's Restaurants while others struck out on their own. "Of course, we have similarities but I think people would be amazed at how diverse we are – thirteen individual identities," said Ed Brengman.

Each brought their own expertise to the table when three of the brothers – Ed, Robert and Gerald – took the dive into the world of wine with the creation of the Brengman Brothers Crain Hill Vineyards. After purchasing land in 2003 and planting twenty acres of vines, the brothers began a quest to make great wines.

They opened their picturesque tasting room in 2011 with a selection of Brengman Brothers Reserve wines, a mid-priced wine list under the Runaway Hen label and in 2012 added a series of Italian imported Refosco wines.

The brothers demonstrated their commitment to creating 'old world' influenced wines by bring the European tradition of celebrating a Feast of St. Vincent to Leelanau in 2013. The patron saint of wine growers and wine makers was honored with a blessing of the vineyards, plenty of good food and of course, plenty of opportunities to sample some Brengman Brothers wine.

Interview with Ed, Robert and Gerald Brengman:

Ed Brengman

How did you gravitate from Detroit to Leelanau to start a winery?

Ed: Robert and Gerald already were living and working here. The area is beautiful and when we made the decision to start a vineyard and eventually a winery, Robert and I started looking. You call it Holy Water and I say it was the Holy Spirit with some divine intervention that brought us here. We were driving up Center Hwy on the peninsula and I spotted a nearly covered realty sign lying in the snow. If I was looking in the other direction I might never have seen it. It was an old fruit orchard and was exactly what we were looking for – two years later we had the hills covered with grape vines.

What inspired the idea of a vineyard?

Ed: Our uncle, Tom Scheuerman, has been growing grapes and making award-winning wines with Bryan Ulbrich on Old Mission peninsula for many years. So we already had excellent mentors. Our first few crops were sent right to Bryan and the resulting wines told us we were definitely on the right track. (Uncle Tom and Bryan of Left Foot Charley Winery won the prestigious Jefferson Cup Invitational for their Riesling in 2012).

You also mentioned being very specific in the selection of grapes grown in certain areas of your property. Is there expansion in the future?

Ed: Yes, it's already started with our purchase of land for the Cedar Lake Vineyard, which we think offers an excellent protected location to grow grapes for red wines. And we've added the Timberly Vineyard – each has its own 'terroir' and uniqueness.

Where did the Runaway Hen label come from?

Ed: We purchase guinea hens each spring and turn them loose in the vineyards to help control the insects. Unfortunately, not all of them return when we round them up every night. Some of them run away, some probably fall prey to predators and maybe some of them end up on the neighbor's dinner table (laughing).

What is your wine philosophy for Brengman Brothers?

Ed: Each of us probably has a bit different philosophy. I just like to drink good quality wine at a reasonable price. So I see that as my philosophy and hope the objective of this winery is to produce good wines that people enjoy and can purchase for good value.

Describe you and your brothers with wine…

Ed: I'm a dry guy and actually the reverse of most people. I'm learning to appreciate the semi-sweet and sweet wines. I guess I'm starting to revert back to those wines I started with in high school (laughing). Robert is whatever wine you want to classify as long as it's sophisticated – he has the true palate in the family. And Gerald, he'll take the grape right off the vine – doesn't even wait for it to be bottled.

Gerald Brengman

If there were such a thing as an ideal growing season for your grapes, what would it be?

Gerald: I don't worry about Mother Nature anymore, I just work with her – as much as you'd like, you can't change her. If I were to get ideal weather it would be hot, dry and long. That would be a VERY extended August in Michigan.

What do you consider your wine philosophy?

Gerald: From my perspective it would be to feed the land – take care of the earth to take care of your vines.

Why do you think the Crain Hill Vineyards location is so special?

Gerald: We sit between a bay and a lake, which gives you an excellent and fairly consistent temperature during the growing season. The growing season itself is extended, which allows the grape to mature and ripen. That means the winemaker can leave the vine alone and let nature take its course.

But you can't just let Nature take its course in growing the grapes, correct?

Gerald: That is one of the surprising things for people to understand about a vineyard. For some reason, many people think you just plant the vines and 'let'em grow.' They don't understand the amount of time invested in each vine. We have 20,000 vines here at Crain Hill and someone spends 5 to 15 minutes with each one every time they're in contact with it and they visit each one checking for disease and overall health many times. That all adds to the cost but it also adds to the quality of the wine as well. It would be easy if you could just let them grow wild (laughing).

For you, what is the most difficult grape to grow?

Gerald: My personal favorite and challenge is the Gewurztraminer grape. It's a pain in the 'you know what' to grow but what a great wine it makes.

Describe you and your brothers with wine...

Gerald: Ed is a bold red and will burst on to your taste buds. Robert is the mystery wine that you can't quite figure out the flavor – an evolving creative wine. Me – I'm all about today – a nice, easy white wine. I'm smooth and good to go.

Robert Brengman

Your brothers acquiesced to your creative nature on the design for the label. Why the pentagon shape?

Robert: It's unique. When we started there were originally five voices or commitments to the project and I wanted the image to reflect that.

Was there any discussion regarding the advantages or pitfalls of having your name on each bottle?

Robert: Do you mean arguments (laughing)? Ironically, we started with just the name Crain Hill Vineyards to identify our location but that kinda backfired when people started to associate us with the $3 jugs of wine made by Crane Lake Winery in California (NOOOO!). When we advanced to become a winery, we settled on the traditional European model of using your last name. But there is a burden and some trepidation with that as well. I occasionally remind my children about the ramifications of negative press having an effect on the family business. Thankful we've been pretty lucky and raised decent kids (laughing).

The bottles are very cool and colorful. Where do they come from?

Robert: The whole concept here is to maximize the experience – getting the people to connect with what we're doing here. The bottles are a part of that. They are made in Germany specifically for the German-type wines: the Rieslings, the Gewurztraminers and so forth. They are traditional but yet unique, especially around here.

Tell us about your Italian wine connection.

Robert: Giovanni Dal Vecchio owns the Valpanera Winery in northern Italy and we connected through a mutual friend who happened to be his college roommate, who I met through work. Valpanera specializes in producing fantastic red wines and wanted to offer their customers some fine white wines – a partnership was formed based on mutual needs.

Describe you and your brothers with wine:
Robert: I'm a Pinot Noir – very difficult to control, takes a lot of nurturing but once it's there, nothing comes close to it – a conversation stopper – in a good way (laughing). Ed is a red – not a straight up Cab but a good Bordeaux blend. Gerald is a Muscat – colorful, a crowd pleaser and fun, with a lot of flavor.

(As I was interviewing Robert at the Festival, Ed came bursting in saying 'come on, what are you, in the middle of confession…get back out here and party!')

I must confess – the Brengman brothers are serious about making good wine but they're just as serious about sharing *La Dolce Vita* **(the good life).** *Grazie, amici mio* **(thank you my friends).**

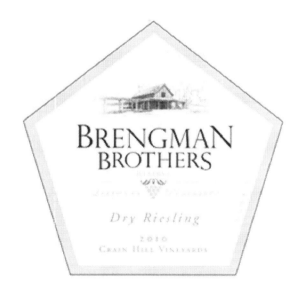

CHATEAU DE LEELANAU
New Owners Bring New Life to Wine

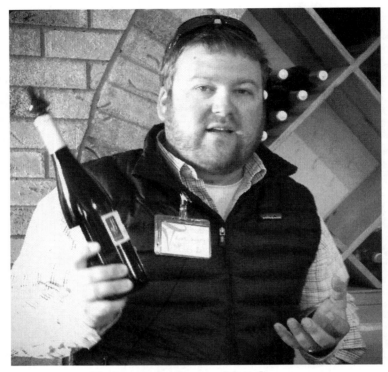

Chateau de Leelanau – Matt Gregory

Chateau de Leelanau has been around since the turn of the century – not that century, the newest one in 2000. After several decades of growing grapes and a decade of making wine, Dr. Roberta Kurtz sold the operation to five guys, most of them her neighbors who were looking for the right fit to get into the wine industry. They took an old brand and made it the 'new kids on the block.'

It all started when Don and Bob Gregory asked Matt Gregory put together a feasibility study for the family business, Cherry Bay Orchards. They were looking to expand into growing wine grapes for local Leelanau wineries. "At the time, my wonderful study went nowhere," Matt laughed. "But it did open my eyes to the potential of growing grapes and making wine."

A few years later, the founding owners of Chateau de Leelanau (who had grown wine grapes since the late '80's and opened the winery in 2000) approached the Gregorys about purchasing their operation. After some discussion and submitting a proposal – *deja vu*, nowhere. The ball got rolling again in 2009 and a purchase agreement was accepted. A partnership was formed with Don Gregory (Matt's uncle and Cherry Bay business owner), Andrew Gregory (Matt's brother), Mark Miezio (cousin and Cherry Bay business partner) and Roger Veliquette (Cherry Bay business partner).

Matt became the Tasting Room manager. "All the other partners are active in other aspects of the company – I had the time and interest to devote to the day to day operations," Matt said. "I discovered it's actually double time…far from the easiest work I've done but easily the most rewarding."

They actually purchased a 'turn-key' operation with a large production facility, a tasting room and 27 acres of mature grapevines with eight different wine grape varietals. That first year, Shawn Walters at French Road Cellars handled the winemaking duties. From then on, it's been theirg 'baby.' "I can honestly tell all our customers that several of us have been on the business end of every drop of wine from the vineyards to the tasting room."

In 2010, the entire operation was handled in-house. Although Matt is officially the general manager, the partners have all assisted from time to time. "They really didn't just throw me to the wolves," Matt said. "Anytime I've needed help with anything, my partners have gladly chipped in – we work well as a team."

It didn't take long for their hard work to show dividends, either. Their expertise in growing quality cherries came through in 2012, when they won the Best of Class in Fruit Wine with their Cherry Wine.

With a newly remodeled tasting room, new labels and new wines, Matt has taken a familiar name and given it a new look – the new Chateau de Leelanau.

Interview with Matt Gregory:

Was there ever consideration to give the winery a new name?

Matt: Our actual corporation name is Chateau de Bay and Chateau de Leelanau is a DBA. We thought long and hard about a name change. Having Leelanau in the name was important and there was strong name recognition already there. The value of the existing brand made the decision to retain it easier.

What do you think is the biggest difference between the original owners and the new operation?

Matt: The biggest difference is the new tasting room. If you haven't visited Chateau de Leelanau in the last three years, you won't recognize the place. The previous owners were off-site and we're there seven days a week, which helps us deal with the day-to-day details. My favorite part of my job is working in the tasting room. It's the most effective evaluation tool to let me know if we're meeting the needs of our customers.

The silhouette of the barn and wine bottle silo is a new creation?

Matt: Yes, we completely rebranded the labels. During the beginning stages of our business plan for the winery, we met in one of our offices and there was a large picture of a barn and silo that we all stared at hundreds of times. One day, one of us said 'that could be our logo – we just need to add a wine bottle topper to the silo.' Our designer did a great job from the rough sketch we gave him.

Tell us the history of the barn/silo/tasting room.

Matt: The Hawkins family originally built that barn back in the early 1900's. It has been used for many different things over the years – a calving barn, a machine shop, an ice cream store, an antique store and probably a few others. When we took over, there was what I call a 'six dumpster' remodeling. I opened it up and put in one of the longest bars on the peninsula – it's about 50 ft. long. We can handle a large crowd – we strive to make sure no one stands in line (laughing).

It looks like there is a color system to your labeling or am I imagining that?

Matt: You noticed – it's working (laughing). There are two different styles of labels. The varietal wines are set with pantone specific colors. The other labels for what I call our 'fun' wines have larger labels and we do whatever colors strike our fancy.

There's a Schaub Farm white wine and a Solem Farm red wine – what's the story there?

Matt: We named those after traditional farm families from the Leelanau peninsula. We also make a Hawkins Red as well. It's a tribute to those folks – I haven't heard any clamoring from the Gregorys yet (laughing).

I see you've advertised a 'world-class' Cherry Wine Sangria. What makes it world class?

Matt: I wish I could tell you but there's a secret ingredient in there. Okay, world class might be a stretch but we sell a ton of it in the summer – easily our most popular wine.

When we first met, you and Roger were collecting some big 'hardware' with the Best of Class trophy for your Cherry Wine. What was that experience like?

Matt: Actually, the Michigan Wine & Spirits Competition is the only tasting event we enter. I'm not against people sending their wines to other contests all over the world – good luck to them and many have done well, bringing back honor and recognition to the Michigan wine industry. But in my mind, the only ones I'm really competing against are my peers here in Michigan. So to win that award was very satisfying. It's fun and exciting but I always say 'don't let a medal tell you that wine is supposed to taste good.'

Prior to 2010, you never had to face a tasting room crowd. How is it going?

Matt: The first day standing behind the bar I had over 100 people come through the doors – talk about jumping right in with both feet. Until then, I spent a lot of time talking to the trees while driving a tractor at night picking cherries – not very good experience at meeting and greeting (laughing). We're busy and I'm having fun so I must be doing something right.

Busy is good, fun is good, with good wine…life is good – thanks Matt.

45 NORTH VINEYARDS AND WINERY
"Wine With A Latitude"

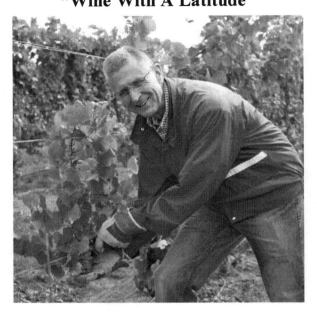

Remember the age-old question – what are friends for? In Steve Grossnickle's case at Forty-Five North…they get you into the business of making wine.

A life-long friend from California planted the seed, so to speak, for Steve to start a winery because 'you can grow vinifera grapes up there.' The 'up there' winery became reality with the purchase of 100 acres of land on the 45th north latitude on the Leelanau peninsula.

Steve was a Navy brat who followed his father in service to his country and working with eyes – dad the optometrist and son the ophthalmologist. "It was great working with my dad," Steve said. "He examined all his friends who needs glasses and sent me all of them who needed cataract surgery (laughing)."

His best friend from sixth grade, Maynard Johnston, is also a doctor in California – pediatrics is his specialty. He also happens to be a part owner in a winery in California and a wine judge at the California State Fair. It was Maynard who steered Steve into winemaking.

"We always joke about a boat being a hole in the water you throw money into," Steve said. "Well, Maynard convinced me to grow grapes here and then I discovered what owning a winery means – it's a tank in which to drown your retirement account (laughing). Now Maynard comes to Michigan twice a year to make sure we're doing things right. Seriously, he's more than a friend - he's a tremendous asset to our business."

After purchasing the property near Lake Leelanau in 2006, the land was tilled and forty acres were planted with grapevines over the next three years. A state-of-the-art production facility was built and award-winning wines began to flow.

Their tasting room is a beautiful barn structure that gives you a 'down home' atmosphere. Just 4,500 miles west of Bordeaux, France, Forty-Five North has its own tradition of producing great wines on the 45th parallel.

Interview with Steve Grossnickle:

The name and logo 45 North comes from being near the 45th parallel, which is where traditional wine regions are – correct?

Steve: We're not just near the 45th parallel...it runs right through our property. My son, Eric designed the logo.

Did that prompt the slogan "Wine on the line"?

Steve: Yes, we had three GPS's all line up just 100 yards south of our tasting room. So, we put a post in the ground with two signs. One says 'Wine on the Line' and below it, another sign says 'Wine with a latitude.' We had a gymnastics team come out last year to practice on the 45th parallel. They wanted to improve their balance...they said it worked (laughing).

Shortly after purchasing your land, you started working with the Leelanau Conservancy. Tell us about that.

Steve: I approached them with a plan to never sell off the winery to developers for housing. When I bought the property, which was owned by local attorney Dean Robb, there were four companies vying for the land to begin housing projects. Dean didn't want to see that happen. Our realtor told us if there were a bidding war, we would have been left in the dust. So, it's really to Dean's credit this land will be preserved.

Your tasting room reflects that preservation attitude as well.

Steve: Originally, we were going to use an antique barn from Wyoming, Michigan that was reassembled on the property but it didn't meet regulations – so it's being used for storage. The new tasting room was built in Ohio by the Amish and reassembled here. For those who haven't been here yet, they can go to Google Maps on their computer and see the facility – just put in 45 North Winery. There are 21 pictures and a 360-degree camera view of inside the tasting room. It's like you are standing right here.

How many 'wine dogs' do you have?

Steve: There are three – a Weimaraner and two Pembroke Welsh corgis. Oh, there's also Alanna's (general manager/daughter-in-law) Golden Retriever, so that's four. Then there's the miniature donkey – so we have at least one 'official' ass running around here too (laughing).

You use a screw cap closure for your wines. Have you gotten any backlash from the traditionalists?

Steve: No, the screw cap has worked fabulously for us.

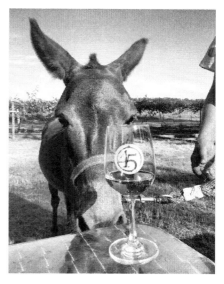

That trend all started basically from New Zealand wineries back in the '80's. There was political turmoil in Portugal, which provides the majority of natural cork for wine bottles. The quality and quantity dropped dramatically and it almost put New Zealand wineries out of business. So they started going to screw caps and use them almost exclusively as their closure now.

You have something rather unusual – a cider made with pears.

Steve: It's a 6.5% alcohol pear cider that is very popular. We also have a traditional hard cider with apples and a 70% apple / 30% cherry cider called Chapple that is doing very well.

What has given you the most satisfaction in owning a winery?

Steve: I would say it's producing quality wines. We are, just as Maynard predicted we could. There are quality wines here and all around Michigan and I'm very proud of that.

Well, I know right where to go to get in perfect balance – thanks Steve.

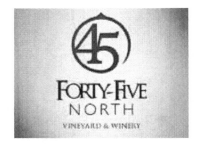

See 45 North's ad on page 393.

GILL'S PIER WINERY
Rocks of the Wine Age

Everyone appreciates something solid – something you can count on. With new wineries opening every year, Gill's Pier Winery has continued to deliver great wines for over a decade on the northern loop of the Leelanau peninsula. How do you find this gem of a winery…look for the rocks.

It was Ryan and Kris Sterkenburg's dream to find a way to live on the peninsula full-time instead of leaving after each visit with

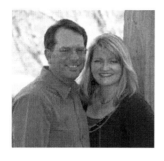

an ache to stay. It was the phenomenal growth in the wine industry that paved the way.

"My in-laws owned property on Leelanau and we always hated to leave," recalled Ryan. "But during each trip we would notice more development, more vineyards and more wineries. We both love wine and started thinking our own winery might be the answer."

Ryan and Kris grew up in Grand Rapids but Ryan's job as a partner in an insurance investment group took the family to Wisconsin. They began asking questions and meeting with various winery owners and vintners. "As our research continued, we realized this was something we wanted to do," Ryan said.

The next thing to do was figure out how to make it happen. "We had some capital and came into the business with open eyes," he said. "We also realized it was going to take a lot of personal sweat equity."

In 2002, the Sterkenburgs began planting grapevines. Two giant rocks were rolled into place, marking the entrance to their new tasting room, which opened in 2003. Gill's Pier Winery became the 13th winery on Leelanau peninsula. "We opened quietly in November of 2003 and the following Memorial Day weekend had a grand opening that became known as the Swine & Dine event."

Now there are 26 wineries represented on the three wine tour loops promoted by the Leelanau Peninsula Vintners Association, with more soon to come. However, Gill's Pier remains one of just a handful of wineries with owners who are actually there doing the work themselves. From late February to harvest time, Ryan is in his own vineyard and assisting his growers with theirs to maintain a consistent, high-quality supply of grapes for his winemaker, Bryan Ulbrich of Left Foot Charley Winery.

With only seven wines in their lineup, Gill's Pier keeps it simple. "I love our wines," Ryan said. "People know what to expect. We want to continue offering great wines that our customers rely on year after year."

Interview with Ryan Sterkenburg:

Okay, what's with the huge rocks and potato wagon at the entrance to your winery?

Ryan: The rocks were my father-in-law's idea – he always had an affinity for large things. He thought people would see them and say 'hey, look at those big rocks – oh, there's a winery here, let's go in. He was right (laughing). The potato wagon also represents his family heritage. It was his father who started the Koeze Nut Company in Grand Rapids and they made deliveries out of a wagon similar to the one that sits out front. That's just one of many antiques at Gill's Pier.

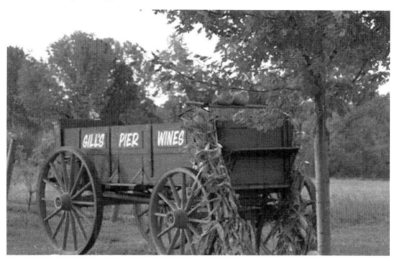

You've incorporated a lot of antiques into the winery's motif. Do you have any favorites?

Ryan: Our favorite is the tasting room bar. It's over 100 years old and was an old trapper's bar from Long Lake, New York in the Adirondack Mountains. We bought it off the internet and the couple actually delivered it to us. The first thing they said was 'we really love this thing, if you don't want it, we'll take it back.' We fell in love with it too. It's 14 ft. long and has beautiful bird's eye maple railing – it's our signature piece. The other piece we love is our Belgian 10 ft. doors that open into our St. Wenceslaus
Room, where we hold special events.

What kind of events do you have in that room?

Ryan: We do private tastings for couples and groups. We also donate a tasting tour to charities for fundraisers. The winning bidder gets a food pairing with several wines, usually I do a 1 ½ hr. presentation on our history and wines. It's a $200 value for a group of eight.

Was there really a place called Gill's Pier?

Ryan: It actually is the historical area where our winery is located. We were originally thinking Pine Hill or Cherry Hill Vineyard but it was my mother-in-law who said 'we're right here in Gill's Pier', the settlement founded by the Bohemians back in the 1800's. There's still a Gill's Pier Road and the St. Wenceslaus Church is referred to as Gill's Pier Church.

Your slogan is 'Where water and wine meet." Could you explain that?

Ryan: We have a beautiful pond out back – it's a great place to have a glass or share a bottle of wine. As the crow flies, we're less than a mile from Lake Michigan. We associate the water and wine with a relaxing and comfortable place. We want people to have a good experience – not emphasizing a wine with certain foods but rather what wine do you like with food. Who doesn't love a picnic by the water with some wine?

How does your label image represent Gill's Pier?

Ryan: We needed to come up with a logo and were throwing out a bunch of ideas. It was my wife Kris who worked with a graphics designer and came up with the water, land, and sun impression. We wanted something that has an association with our location in an artistic manner – everyone loved it so we've stuck with it.

There has to be a story behind your Royce, Whitewater and Unleashed wines.

Ryan: The one thing about those three wines is consistency – no matter what the blend, they will always represent our dry white, sweet white and dry red wines. Royce comes from the Auxerrois grape (pronounced oh zher WAH) we used one year and no one knew how to say it – it kept coming out OX ah royce, so we gave up and just started calling it Royce. The Houdek Dunes are located right across the street and owned by the Leelanau Conservancy. We contracted to donate a portion of the proceeds to them with our Houdek Creek Whitewater Wine, which eventually became just Whitewater Wine. And the Just Unleashed Wine was a wild untamed red wine that reminded us of our wine dogs running around and the need to tame them. Just Unleashed seemed appropriate.

Tell us about your Swine and Dine event.

Ryan: My father-in-law again suggested having a big pig roast as a grand opening event in 2004. So we decided to have it on Memorial weekend. It was free and open to the public – a nice coming out party. It went over so well, we decided to do it every year. It's still free - we've added live music and use the event to introduce our new releases for the year. Most of all, we use it as a way to say thank you to our loyal customer base.

I know the winery has been up for sale but what's next for you and Gill's Pier?

Ryan: We'll carry on until the right buyer comes along. Our kids were in the 2nd grade and kindergarten when we moved up here and now they're in college. So we'd like to spend more 'adult' time with them. We feel and hope we've created a great brand and someone comes in with the same passion we've had for wine – someone who will maintain the quality then make their own mark by growing Gill's Pier to a new level.

It will be a tough act to follow and they better not move the rocks – thanks Ryan.

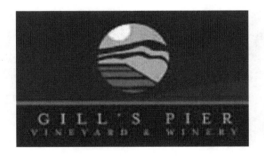

GOOD HARBOR WINERY
Good Wine, Good Times, Good People

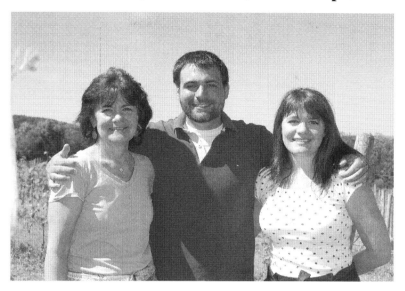

Bruce Simpson was a legend in the Michigan wine industry. Sadly, 'the gentle giant' passed away in 2009 but his impact is still being felt. He left behind many good things. The best is the family team – his wife, son and daughter - that still operates the Good Harbor Winery on the Leelanau peninsula near the village of Leland.

Debbie, his college sweetheart and wife of nearly thirty-one years, still manages the tasting room and handles the label design; Sam is the winemaker and operations manager and Taylor manages Sales Distribution and Marketing. Together, they are continuing to nurture the Simpson legacy that began as the fourth winery on the peninsula.

Bruce's father, the founder of the Harbor Hill Fruit Farms, had already predicted the decline in the wholesale cherry market as Bruce was graduating from Michigan State with a degree in agriculture. They were looking to diversify so Bruce went on to the University of California at Davis to learn the wine business. He and Debbie returned in 1978, got married and began building Good Harbor Winery, which opened its doors in 1980.

"If Bruce were here, I'm sure he'd say he learned a lot more doing the winemaking than he ever did sitting in a classroom," Debbie said. "It's so expensive to get a winery started but at least we already had the land. We remodeled the tasting room quite a few years ago and Bruce said that cost more than it did to build laughing)."

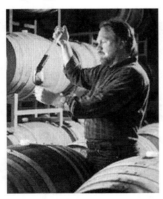
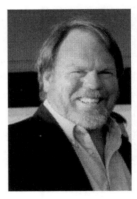

With their father's passing, the children returned to the peninsula. The decision was made after one year to lease the Harbor Hill orchards and concentrate on running the winery. "I think their passion is in the wine business," Debbie said. "They saw their father build something good and put thirty years into the business – they want it to live on."

With the help of neighboring winemakers like Larry Mawby and Lee Lutes, the transition was smooth and successful. Bruce's legacy has continued on with the second generation. He would be proud to know Good Harbor Winery is still in good hands.

Interview with Debbie Simpson:

The parent company is Harbor Hill Fruit Farm – so why not Harbor Hill Winery?

Debbie: The whole operation, with over three hundred and fifty acres of orchards and 65 acres of vineyards, is right across from Good Harbor. We liked the name Good Harbor Winery and that's where we are located.

What makes Good Harbor Winery unique?

Debbie: We started Good Harbor with the idea of producing quality wines at a reasonable price – so people could afford to drink our wine on more than just a special occasion. Now that the kids are involved, we actually have a more diverse range of wines and it's nice to offer more choices.

Has there been a philosophy behind the winemaking at Good Harbor?

Debbie: I'd say we always tried to keep it simple and give the customer what they want. I'm basing that on our three most popular wines, which are Trillium, Fishtown and Harbor Red – all blends. We originally tried to sell the wines by their hybrid names, like Seyval, Marechal Foch, or Vignoles. Nobody knew what they were or how to pronounce them and it didn't work.

The other factor is we're a family operation – people know this and that atmosphere comes through when they're here. I think people like that about us.

Good Harbor Winery was #4 on the peninsula. Tell us about the first three.

Debbie: The first was Bernie Rink at Boskedyl. He is brilliant and had the vision to start this whole thing up here. He's also a very nice guy but he won't let everyone know that (laughing). I really don't know much about Leelanau Cellars other than they started around the same time that we did. And Larry Mawby has been a good friend for so long. He and Bruce started the first vineyard management company up here and were very successful. He was right there to help Sam as well after Bruce passed.

What was your first big hit with the wines?

Debbie: I'd say it was Trillium. Bruce had a vision of what he wanted our label to look like (a pencil sketch of the tasting room). One day we went into a wine shop in Grand Rapids back in the early 80's and there was one Good Harbor bottle on the bottom shelf all covered with dust…we both agreed we needed a new label. Our next blend needed a name. I spotted some flowering Trillium by the road on the way to Mackinaw and said let's call it Trillium. We had a graphic designer put a Trillium flower with a pink background on the label. It really popped and got us on our way.

With your art education background, are you the 'art critic' for label design?

Debbie: I'm not the art critic – I just pick what I like (laughing). I have my favorite artists and usually commission them to create our vision for the label. Our Pinot Grigio Reserve label was one of my grandmother's paintings, which hangs in my living room. Bruce spotted a painting of Fishtown in a friend's house, which we used for the Fishtown White label.

Do you pick the picture and create the wine or create the wine then find the picture?

Debbie: Actually, it's worked both ways. Most of the time it involves sitting around the table with a bottle of wine brainstorming. My daughter has a black Labrador named Betty, so I suggested naming our new Cabernet based blend, Labernet. We had another red blend that we decided to name Collaboration with my friend's quilt on the label. Each label has a story.

You've worked in the tasting room for many years…what is the strangest thing you've ever been asked?

Debbie: As I've said, Fishtown is one of our popular wines and Fishtown is a charming historic fishing village just down the road. It's actually Leland but all the locals still refer to it as Fishtown. I can understand when someone says 'Fishtown – that's an unusual name for a wine' but when someone asks if there really is fish in the wine – that's strange. I've also been asked what the cherry wine is made of, which always makes me chuckle.

What's the biggest difference between Bruce and Sam as winemakers?

Debbie: Bruce had to learn so much by trial and error. Sam graduated from MSU with a degree in finance, so he approaches the business with a different business perspective. A good example is Sam had the idea to convert many of our vineyard operations over to machinery, which is a huge labor saving device and wasn't available in Bruce's time. The machinery allows us to manage our own vineyards in a fraction of the time and also has allowed us to offer the service to neighboring vineyards. With proper vineyard management, you can still keep the grape quality high without hand picking – it's amazing.

An explanation is needed concerning the family dynamics during the Big Ten football season. Bruce, Sam and you graduated from MSU. Taylor graduated from the U of M. But you also were born and raised in Columbus, Ohio, the home of Ohio State. How does the family handle these rivalries?

Debbie: When Michigan plays OSU, I root for the Buckeyes. Unfortunately, Taylor is outnumbered, so when MSU plays Michigan, she just leaves and watches the game somewhere else. I totally understand a divided household.

What wine best represents you?

Debbie: Oh, my children call me 'the Chardonnay Queen' and I've earned it (laughing).

I'll go with Taylor (fellow Michigan grad) and my wife (MSU) can stay with you but as the Collaboration continues, Good Harbor Winery will thrive – thanks Debbie.

See Good Harbor's ad on page 405.

LARRY MAWBY
Conquering The Sparkling Wine World

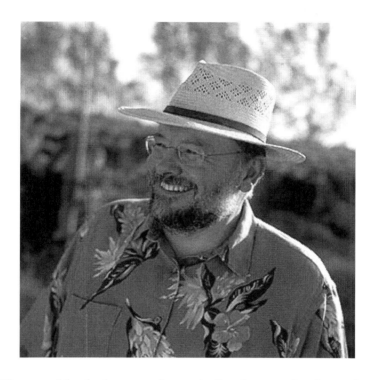

When you blend a boy growing up in the cherry orchards south of Suttons Bay, with an English major college graduate, and then add an expert in making sparkling wine, you get the one and only Larry Mawby. Since he planted his first grape vines in 1973, Larry has carved a niche and become a genuine 'character' in the Michigan wine industry.

The Mawby tradition of fruit growing began with his grandfather's peach and apple orchards in the Rockford area. Then his father bought a cherry orchard on the Leelanau

Peninsula in 1953 and Larry eventually managed the family farm until he opened the tasting room of L. Mawby Vineyards in 1978.

"At that time, there were only three wineries up here – Boskydel, Leelanau Cellars and Chateau Grand Traverse," said Larry. "No one had a clear picture of what varieties would grow well or even what consumers would want to buy." His first wine was called Picnic Rosé, which was a pink wine 'with all the grapes put together.'

The decision to concentrate solely on sparkling wines using the champagne method was made in 1996, and then, in 2004, he added the M. Lawrence brand.

Although, there are more wineries in Michigan making sparkling wines, there still is only one Larry Mawby.

Interview with Larry Mawby:

How many people told you that sparkling wines couldn't be made in northern Michigan?

Larry: I don't know because I never asked anybody. You have to remember back then there wasn't a norm, there was barely the notion of growing grapes for wine up north – it was still very questionable. That's why there were only four wineries for nearly a decade. Everyone was waiting for one of us to fail.

So what eventually steered you in the direction of making just sparkling wines?

Larry: It was a logical consequence of looking at the grape varieties that grow well here and determining those grapes could make a nice sparkling wine and be reliable every year. As Clint Eastwood said in Magnum Force, 'a man's got to know his limitations.' For me, it was realizing I couldn't make both table wines and sparkling wines and be the best at either one. When there were only a dozen wineries up here, people couldn't visit them all in one trip and now there are more than 30, so it's even worse – people have to make choices. We're working on getting the message out – if you come through our tasting room doors, I sure hope you're looking for sparkling wines (laughing).

Is the process of making table wines and sparkling wines very different?

Larry: At the heart, winemaking is pathetically simple – you break the skin of the berry and yeast starts consuming the sugar, producing alcohol; you separate the solids and liquids – wine; let it go – vinegar. With sparkling wine, you capture the CO_2 from fermentation to create another fermentation. Actually, you grow the grapes different and really, looking at the process holistically, everything is different.

Your Talisman Brut appeared in The Great Wines of America book. Has that wine won you the most awards?

Larry: No, actually we've done as well with several wines in competitions. I'm not a big fan of wine competitions. They serve two purposes – as an ego-stroker for the winemaker or winery owner and they're useful for marketing. But they don't say anything about the quality of the wines. I appreciate the awards but it's not reality.

Why is that?

Larry: What winning means is on that day, that group of tasters favored that wine. Take the same group, the next day they'll probably pick a different wine. Take a different group the same day and they'll probably pick a different wine. A judge might be trying 300 different wines and most people's palate fatigues after 30 or 40 – so, even the order they taste them is a factor. The true test is producing a quality wine that people enjoy year after year.

It says L. Mawby on the label, which in itself puts a little more pressure on the winemaker. Why did you decide to put your moniker on the label?

Larry: I thought about it a lot and ultimately, I decided if I was going to be serious about making wines, I would put my name out there. But it wasn't an ego thing or a smart marketing tool either – people couldn't pronounce it and kept saying 'what's an L. Mawby?' (laughing).

Do the names of your wines reflect your personality?

Larry: They all are a part of me, so, yes they reflect my personality. But there are a number of different explanations for the concept of a wine's name. Sometimes it's a characteristic of the wine. Sometimes you have a name and the wine is created to assume that role. Some are whimsical and some are traditional. The true art of winemaking is when you make a wine that tastes like its name.

What is the primary difference between the L. Mawby wines and the M. Lawrence wines?

Larry: The L. Mawby wines are bottle-fermented and take two or three years to come out for sale. The M. Lawrence wines are tank fermented and are ready in months.

If you were the czar of the wine industry, what would you do?

Larry: Well, considering the aspiration for our wine is world domination, I'm stunned by the potential (laughing). Seriously, I would make the 3-tier system optional instead of mandatory...but I would also make daily wine consumption mandatory as well (laughing).

Actually, that doesn't surprise me at all...thanks Larry.

ONE WORLD WINERY
The Wide World of Wines With Shawn Walters

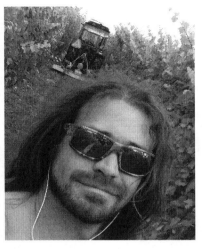

As a teenager, Shawn Walters had visions of being a professional snowboarder. That career was put on hold when he entered the world of winemaking. In less than a decade, Shawn reached the top of the wine world with multiple international Best of Show awards in some of the most prestigious wine competitions.

Now one of the most sought after winemakers, Shawn has always had an 'all-in' type of personality with a chip on his shoulder. "I'm passionate about what I do and good at it and plan on making the best wines possible until I die," he said. "I've even got a Riesling tattoo, man, I'm committed." His rise to prominence started like most winemakers – as a 'cellar rat.'

A native of the Traverse area, Shawn was a seasonal worker – chairlift operator/snowboarder in the winter and a cook at the Riverside Inn the rest of the year. His commitment to detail started him on a new career path. "Bill Skolnick, the head winemaker for Leelanau Cellars, liked his chicken done a certain way and I cooked it for him," Walters recalled. "One day he offered me a job at the winery. It was full-time, with benefits – I was young and figured if it didn't work out, I could always do something else."

That was in the fall of 1993 and he started to learn winemaking, literally from the ground up. After five years, Shawn left to help winemaker Lee Lutes start the Black Star Farms wine operation. "That was an awesome experience," he said. "They were purchasing all new equipment - I watched a winery being built and learned a lot working with Lee."

In 2000, Leelanau Cellars hired Shawn back – this time as the head winemaker and vineyard manager. Under his watch, they went from 35,000 cases to over 100,000 cases sold annually. Walters also began helping smaller wineries get a toehold in the industry. Within a few years, he was bringing Alan Eaker's Longview Winery international acclaim with several Best of Show wines.

Then it was on to help 45 North launch a new winery in 2007. With their first few vintages, Walters was again producing award-winning wines. After racking up multiple Best of Class and double-gold awards in competitions from the Finger Lakes region of New York to the Pacific Rim with different wineries, Shawn opened his own business in 2009 called One World Winery Consulting.

His focus remains on working with smaller 'boutique' wineries that make estate-grown artisan wines. "I don't have any formal training in winemaking," Shawn said. "I learned by being a cellar rat extraordinaire. I watched and learned from Bill and Lee, then got my degree from the school of hard knocks. I'm pretty hard-headed too (laughing)."

Based out of Doug Mathies' French Road Cellars and their custom crush facility, Walters is currently making wines for more than a half-dozen wineries in northern Michigan.

Interview with Shawn Walters:

When you are working with different vineyard/winery owners, how much input do they have in the finished product?

Shawn: First, we discuss what grows best with their land or *terroir*. Then we discuss what they want the end result to be. Throughout the growing season, I'm in contact with them managing the vineyard based on the growing season we're experiencing. Then we get ramped up for the harvest. We can crop the vineyard according to the style we've decided on. For instance, you crop Pinot Noir different if you want to use the grapes for a Rosé or if it will be a red wine. An owner has a lot of say in the finished result.

I've heard the phrase 'it's all about the balance.' What does that mean?

Shawn: I'm not a big fan of manipulating the chemistry of the juice. Once the grapes have been crushed and I look at the chemistry, then I pick a yeast based on what the customer wants. As the fermentation process works, you may have to do some enzyme or temperature adjustments based on the fruit you're working with. But the ultimate 'balance' is when the whole process works naturally. The question becomes 'do we have to do something or can we leave it alone and let it become what it is?' More times than not, those are your best wines.

What factors do you use to determine bottling time?

Shawn: That's a whole other game in the wine process. Part of my consulting with clients is to ask questions like 'can you afford to hold on to a red in barrels for two years or do you need a quick turn around and have the wine drinkable in 10 months?' With whites, does the person want to sit on it for six months or based on their current inventory, do we need to bottle sooner, etc. Personally, I like to bottle earlier with whites to capture the essence of the young fruit – many winemakers think it's premature but I've had a lot of success with that method. There's passion in winemaking but there's also the bottom line to consider.

Is there a difference in your winemaking from those Leelanau Cellars days and now?

Shawn: Actually, there's very little difference. What I wanted to do was to raise the bar in this area. I wanted to make clean vibrant wines that consumers really enjoy – wines that are varietally expressive and correct. That's what I wanted then and that's what I still try to do with each vintage.

What's the biggest difference in the Michigan wine industry from twenty years ago?

Shawn: The fruit growers are listening to winemakers more now. They're getting the proper yields and improving the quality of fruit – keeping the diseases down and still being environmental friendly. There's also a lot of cooperation and exchange of information to improve the quality of wine.

Does your wine style differ greatly from other winemakers?

Shawn: I do the very best I can in doing what the client wants, which might not be what I would do personally. I don't know how much my style differs from others but I have certain ways of doing things. We do everything very gentle – no aggressive agitation that might promote bitterness; a cool fermentation and checked twice a day. I would say my style is producing clean, crisp, fresh, young wine.

What is the big difference between producing a Michigan red wine and white wine?

Shawn: They are completely separate animals. The biggest difference is the quality based on the climate we have to deal with here. We can make some of the best white wines in the world. That's not me saying it – that's international sommeliers. Our Rieslings rival anyone's, period. As far as red wines go, even from a great growing season like 2012, it's tough to make a red that competes internationally. Having said that, we still occasionally win golds, double golds and Best of Class with our reds. Michigan just isn't getting the respect in the national or international wine journals. Reds are just tougher all around, in growing and vineyard management but especially money wise. You've got $6 per bottle just in the barrel expense for a good Pinot Noir.

You have won many Best of Class/Best of Show awards – what do you think sommeliers are tasting in your wines that has made them stand out?

Shawn: They want the wine to taste correct, i.e. a Riesling should taste like a Riesling. They want balance, i.e. the right ratio of acid, PH and sugar. And they want the wine to be clean with no apparent winemaking flaws. But to pick out any one thing they're getting from my wines...I haven't got a clue. I wish I knew so I could do that with every wine I make (laughing).

When it comes to vineyard management and winemaking, what's the best piece of advice you've gotten?

Shawn: Doug Mathias of French Road Cellars told me 'if you really want to do something special you have to stay on it.' By that, he meant it's an every day, hands on task so you know what's going on all the time. You and only you can make it happen by staying on it. He's right.

Take six highly respected winemakers with the same equipment and the same high quality fruit – what is the end result?

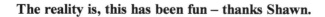

Shawn: You will get six distinctly different wines. They will probably all be good wines but some or maybe none will be gold medal winners because of the subjective nature of competitions. It would make a fun reality show, wouldn't it?

The reality is, this has been fun – thanks Shawn.

WILLOW VINEYARDS & WINERY
When A Dream Comes True

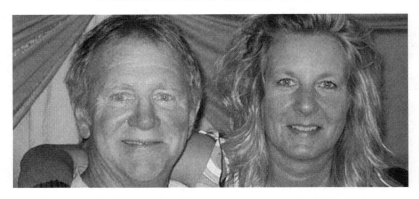

When John and Jo Crampton were newly married, which has been over 35 years now, it was a romantic hillside picnic during an adventure through the Leelanau peninsula that changed their lives forever. "We sat talking about the marvelous view and dreamed about owning a place like this," John recalled. That dream would become reality and eventually became their vineyard and Willow Winery.

"Call it fate or destiny or whatever, but we literally walked over a fallen Coldwell Banker For Sale sign coming down the hill," he said. "We wrote down the telephone number, then we had to find a payphone – it was way before cell phones (laughing)."

They made the call, they made an offer and became the proud owners of their dream hillside by the next weekend. John was a professional landscaper for his family's business. He and Jo also operated nurseries to supply landscaping jobs in southeast Michigan. But the pull to return to Leelanau was too much and they soon moved there permanently nearly thirty years ago.

"My grandfather ran a summer camp near the Mesick/Buckley area and I knew from a young age that I wanted to live up north," John said. "A few years after getting the property we moved into a small cottage on the bay – we knew nothing about the wineries up here and at the time there were only four on the peninsula."

How many times have you heard 'well, it all started when I had this dream'? It was somewhere around eight years after moving north when the Cramptons decided to plant wine grapes on their hillside property and John had that dream. "One night I dreamt I went to work for Larry Mawby at the L. Mawby Winery and a few weeks later I stopped in to tell him about it...he hired me (laughing)."

John learned the winemaking craft under Mawby's tutelage for four years while they continued to nurture their own vineyard. After a few vintages were bottled, the fledgling vintner left the nest and they opened the Willow Winery tasting room in 1998.

With eight acres in vines, Willow Winery features five estate wines that are sold exclusively in the tasting room. The groomed vineyard provides a picturesque view on one side and out the front visitors still have the spectacular view of Grand Traverse Bay that John and Jo dreamed about at the very beginning of this adventure.

Interview with John Crampton:

Coming from a landscaping background, what are you most proud of at Willow Winery?

John: I designed and built nearly everything here. The house and tasting room were placed in the hillside instead of on top and we look out over eighteen miles of water. The tasting room is literally on the edge of the vineyard. It's a place people just want to walk through and be a part of, which we encourage.

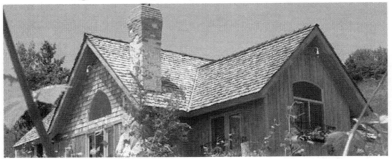

You got started with Larry Mawby, now your winemaker is Chris Guest. How did you guys get hooked up?

John: We've known each other since we were twenty and eighteen. We actually had a softball team together called the Roosters – I think we were 2 –34 but fortunately we're better winemakers than softball players. He's been making wine for more than 30 years and was the head winemaker for the Seven Lakes Winery in Fenton before moving up here. There are a lot of things that have to be done right for the wine to be right and you only have one vintage a year to work with. We work well together.

Tell us how you came up with the name Willow Winery.

John: There was a giant majestic willow tree down at the end of our driveway. Unfortunately, it was badly damaged in an ice storm one year and I had to take it down. But we decided to name the vineyard and winery after it. The whole naming process started as a tug of war between Jo and me. She wanted to name the place Thistle Bay. I finally convinced her otherwise when I told her to imagine how difficult it would be to say Thistle Bay after three or four glasses of wine. She finally agreed.

There are a lot of antiques & pictures in the tasting room – any favorites?

John: We have a nice collection of die-casts, lithographs and prints – our centerpiece, from 1896, is a beautiful lady holding a glass of Rosé. People just love looking at her and the rest of the collection.

You have chosen to have a wine cat named Frankie...

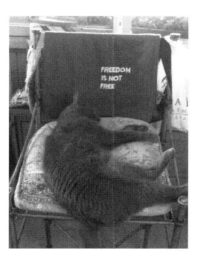

John: He's a Brooklyn cat so you pronounce his name FranKEE. He takes pleasure in running up the vineyard pole on occasion and sit up there like a crow surveying his territory. Frankie's a fixture around here and the people love him. We don't have dogs because we go south in the winter for a while and the cat doesn't need all that attention – except when he demands to get his morning scratch.

There are two wines on your list called Pretty In Pink and Sweet Rain – what's their story?

John: Pretty In Pink is a Pinot Noir Rosé that used to be called Baci Rosé, which means kiss in Italian. First, the people would ask what it means and then they'd ask if I was Italian. We gave up about six years ago and changed the name. Sweet Rain is the only real sweet wine we've made. It started with a very unripe vintage of Chardonnay that came from another vineyard. There was so much acidity we just kept pouring the sugar to it and Jo came up with the Sweet Rain name. It's a big seller for us.

You mentioned Larry Mawby being a mentor – did he give you any parting advice?

John: Larry is a great friend and teacher but he gave no parting advice. He just said 'you'll be so busy doing your own thing you won't have time to come back and work for me.' He was SO right (laughing).

What would the John Crampton of today tell John back in 1992?

John: He'd say 'hang in there brother, you'll get there. Put you're best foot forward – the harder you work the luckier you'll get.'

There have been quite a few small weddings at Willow – any surprises?

John: Jo had one pre-wedding surprise. A young man asked her to videotape something in the tasting room. He showed her how to work the camera and then got down on one knee to propose to his girlfriend. Jo was surprised as anyone and you can hear her say 'oh !@#$' on the tape. He left it in and every time they come to visit, we all have a good laugh.

Willow Winery was up for sale – what does the future hold for you and the winery?

John: When we put the winery on the market, it was very poor timing economically. We put so much energy into getting the business going, there wasn't much thought put into an exit strategy. A few years ago, we thought we might be ready to move on to another adventure but the fact is we love living here. It's been a great run but we still love what we're doing and so we'll continue for a while longer and see what happens. As of today, the winery is not for sale.

Well, here's a big thank you for sharing your dream, your view and your wines with us.

> I ran my first 10K today. Just kidding,
> I'm on my third glass of wine.

NORTHWEST - Other

CADILLAC..119
FOX BARN...124
HARBOR SPRINGS....................................129
HEAVENLY VINEYARDS..........................134
LEFT FOOT CHARLEY.............................140
NORTHERN NATURAL.............................146

I'm having fruit salad for dinner. Well, it's mostly grapes.
Ok, it's all grapes. – fermented grapes.
I'm having wine for dinner.

CADILLAC WINERY
Wine 101

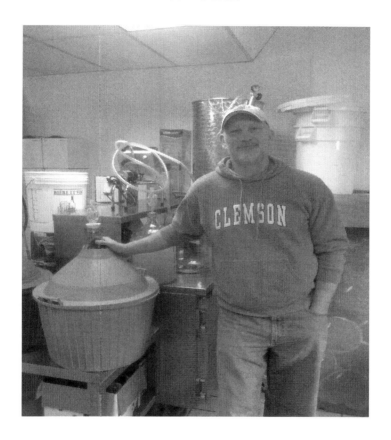

Not to be confused with a freshman class on making wine, Cadillac Winery was the 101st winery licensed in Michigan. However, winemaker Kevin Leahy admits to making a few freshman mistakes along the way. "The first time I won Best of Class at the Michigan State Fair with a cherry dessert wine, I used super ripe cherries and added too much sugar," laughed Kevin.

A Bay City native, Kevin remembers seeing many barrels of wine in the basements of both sets of grandparents. "There is a family rumor that my great grandfather survived the Depression doing a bit of bootlegging and selling wine by the glass," admitted Leahy.

He started a home wine and brew kit business with the intent of reviving those family winemaking traditions. "It has almost become a lost art that was passed from generation to generation," said Kevin. "The first time I took six wines to the state fair I won three gold, two silver and a bronze - it was great confirmation from wine authorities other than just my friends saying 'this is good stuff.'

That validation became the seeds for the Cadillac Winery to open in 2013 just east of the Tustin exit 168 off US 131 and 11 miles south of Cadillac. Travel another 5 miles south and you can see the southern hillsides of the Leahy Rock Vineyard where Kevin tends to the vines that are producing future vintages of Michigan wines.

The freshman winemaker has now graduated and currently the Cadillac Winery is offering 10 selections, including several of Kevin's award-winning wines.

Interview with Kevin Leahy:

How big is Leahy Rock Vineyards and why Leroy, Michigan?

Kevin: It's an 80-acre plot that my great-great-grandmother homesteaded. My father bought it in the '70s and we traveled up there every weekend to build a three-bedroom cabin. Back then I hated it, now I hate leaving. I took 20 acres of the wonderful southern exposed hills for the vineyard. Currently 8 acres are fenced in and five are planted with different varietals.

One of your award-winning wines is called the Glen Grape Zinger - tell us about that.

Kevin: I won the semi dry red category five years in a row with that wine at the Michigan State Fair - that is my secret weapon in the big scheme of the Cadillac Winery (laughing). I saw this small grape patch growing on the way to the cabin and I finally stopped in one day to asked about it. That vine grows like a weed and produces great big blue grapes. I took it up to the MSU Research Center in Leelanau and they don't know what it is. My friend Glen owned the property and planted the vines - Zinger was the name of the original owner, thus Glen Grape Zinger. I've got nearly 2 rows growing at my vineyard right now.

Why Leahy Rock Vineyard?

Kevin: I'm trying to grow grapes there, not rocks. I'm cursed with finding a rock in practically every hole I dig on that land (laughing).

Where did the vision for the Vineyard come from?

Kevin: After college I started experimenting with the home made wines and I would sit up there on the hills during deer hunting season and could visualize rows of grape vines growing there. After my Zinger won at the state fair, I took some old chain-link fence and planted those vines in a 20 x 20 plot - in one year it was bursting through. That's when I knew it would really work.

They say hindsight is 20/20, so would you do anything different?

Kevin: Yes, I should have put all of our energy into getting the tasting room in Leroy up and going first and then start developing the vineyard. Instead, I tried to do both at the same time and there aren't enough hours in the day.

How did you find the building for your tasting room in Leroy?

Kevin: We had several locations picked out that never came to fruition for various reasons. Then a few years ago we went to a tax auction in Clare that had several properties in it from Osceola County. One was a building called Mama Rose's Pizzeria. It has easy access from US 131 and M-115 and is just a few miles from the vineyard. I got the bid on the last nickel we could afford to spend when the gavel fell - so I guess it was meant to be.

How many vines are currently planted in the vineyard and how much do they cost?

Kevin: We currently have about 2600 vines planted, with a focus on Pinot Gris, Riesling, Cab Franc and Pinot Noir. We went to three different nurseries for the rootstock and the prices ranged from $250-$375 for bunches per 100. We take all those nice straight rows for granted out in the fields but if you're a greenhorn farmer like me, it ain't that easy (laughing).

Being so close to Cadillac makes sense for the name of your winery - was that your first choice?

Kevin: No, it was about the fifth choice (laughing). If you look at the landscape of the vineyard, you can see the twin peaks and I was thinking of all the ways you could market that... but ALL the women in my life squelched that idea. Then there was Rose Vineyards - my great-great-grandmother's name was Rose, down the road is Rose Lake, Rose Lake Township, and the Rose golf course but it seemed a little fluffy for me. The vineyard is practically surrounded by groves of beautiful pines so we thought maybe Evergreen Winery but one Google search axed that - Evergreen Chiropractic, Evergreen Septic, Evergreen Plumbing, Evergreen everything! I thought we'd never get the Cadillac Winery name, but we sent in a label application and it came back APPROVED!

We are so glad it was approved - thanks Kevin.

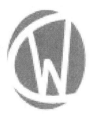

See Cadillac Winery's ad on page 398.

THE FOX BARN WINERY
It's Odd But In A Good Way

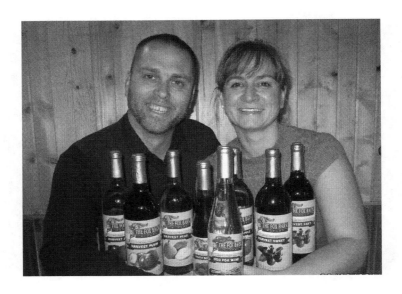

Todd Fox and Kellie Chase grew up in competing farm families and attended rival high schools. It's not the Romeo & Juliet story of Oceana County...but they did get married. Todd took over the Fox Farm operation (1700 acres of fruit trees) and after two children, Kellie opened a farm market and started the Fox Barn Winery. It features among other good wines – Odd Fox Wine made from asparagus (story to follow).

Kellie went back to college but wasn't sure of her career path. "I've never been a 9 to 5er," Kellie said. "I was raised on a farm just like Todd and he finally suggested I should start a farm stand."

She and the kids built their stand out of grower boxes next to a family-owned barn on a busy road near the Silver Lake Sand

Dunes in 2005. That barn would evolve into Fox Barn Marketplace and Winery. "I kept begging Todd to let us use the barn so we didn't have to bring everything in each night. I carved out more space each season and finally after the third year he gave in and I took it over."

In 2007, the idea of a winery came to light. "I actually overheard Todd telling a friend about opening a winery – that was news to me," chuckled Kellie. "I instantly loved the idea."

In 2008, they sold their first bottle of wine and added the tasting room in the barn. The asparagus wine came along in 2010 and now the Fox Barn Winery has a list featuring nine wines and several hard ciders.

But it's the Odd Fox Wine that everyone talks about.

Interview with Kellie Fox:

Was there ever any consideration to calling the winery anything other than Fox Barn?

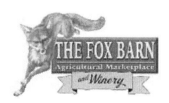

Kellie: I thought about trying to incorporate my maiden name in there somehow, which is Chase. But that big old barn has always had the Fox name on the side – calling it Fox Barn just simplified things.

Your logo of a fox certainly fits the name.

Kellie: That fox comes from a fruit crate label that the Fox family business had in the 1950's. We spruced him up a bit but he's been around a long time.

What's the story behind the trucks out front?

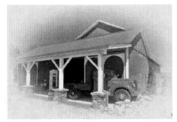

Kellie: We started with a 1947 Diamond T (which came from the Diamond T Motor Company – eventually becoming the Diamond Reo Company) in the barn and sold the wine out of it. But I needed more store space for other things and the truck couldn't hold enough wine anymore. So we moved it outside and added a couple more Diamond T trucks to the display. The Fox family has a trucking company that hauls fruit all across Michigan and they've always had a prestigious fleet of Diamond T's. Those three trucks have been retired – they all still run and no, they're not for sale. People are stopping all the time to ask.

Did you have to do a lot to convert the barn into a marketplace and winery?

Kellie: We called in a great barn restorer to work on it. We had to level the original floor and put a new one in over top. There is lots of new lighting, new plumbing with sinks and new bathrooms – all needed to get certified. So many people remember farming relatives from their childhood and just walk around here remembering – and so many of the children have never even been in a barn before. The barns around the countryside are slowly disappearing.

Is it safe to say you were the first to make asparagus wine?

Kellie: We might not be the first to make it but we're the first, to my knowledge, to sell it commercially. There is someone in Traverse City who is making asparagus beer. We know our asparagus wine is a novelty but I make more of it every year and it keeps selling.

Tell us how Fox Barn came to make asparagus wine.

Kellie: In 2009, Todd brought in a bucket of mashed up asparagus and told me to 'make something of it.' Of course, my first thought was it couldn't possibly taste good! I put the sugar in for fermentation and added yeast. I love asparagus but to be honest it smelled terrible. I put it into a barrel and then off to the side, figuring I'd just be throwing it away in the fall. It came out fairly clear – smelled and tasted like asparagus but we all said 'Wow, this isn't too bad!'

How does the public respond to it?

Kellie: Obviously, if you start out not liking asparagus, this wine won't change your mind. But for those that like asparagus and try it – they react just like we did and say 'this isn't too bad.' That's not the best tag line (laughing) but don't knock until you've tried it.

And who came up with the name, Odd Fox Wine?

Kellie: That would be Todd – I guess when he was a kid they called him Odd Todd.

It sounds to me like you should be winning Best of Class for

vegetable wine in the future.

Kellie: We're having fun with it and the public is too – they're at least curious. The big question seems to be 'does it make your urine smell like asparagus?' I guess some people, after eating enough asparagus, have that issue. To me, it's a sipping wine because of the sugar level, so I tell people if they're inclined to drink the whole bottle in one sitting, let me know (laughing). Maybe we should take a Facebook poll.

You're making tree fruit wine – you've got a pretty good source of fruit – but you're also starting to make more wine from wine grapes. Do you have plans to make estate wines?

Kellie: I've already made small batches (45 cases) of a sweet white blend and a dry red blend – those sold out quickly. We've already planted wine grapes right around the barn and will have a good supply in a few years. It's been a learning curve with wine grapes but Todd has accepted the challenge.

So is there another mystery wine out there for you to discover?

Kellie: I'm not actively looking for one but my husband thinks we should be featuring an entire Odd Fox Wine Series. We are in Oceana County, which is considered the asparagus capital of the world and we've already cornered that market. But I keep telling him we're not doing every vegetable under the sun!

Truthfully, I'm not a fan of asparagus unless my wife puts enough cheese on it but I AM gonna try that wine – thanks Kellie.

See Fox Barn's ad on page 404.

HARBOR SPRINGS VINEYARDS AND WINERY
Through The Trees a Vineyard Appears

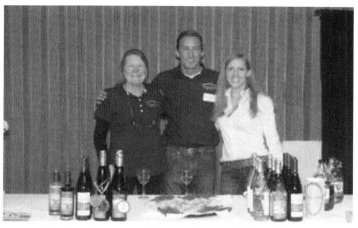

Harbor Springs – Sharon, Jimmy, Marci Spencer

Remember the old axiom 'you can't see the forest for the trees?' Jimmy Spencer saw a vineyard on a forested hillside in the middle of his family's farm called Pond Hill in Harbor Springs. It was an image that became the Harbor Springs Winery in 2010.

Jimmy was a kid from Chicago until his dad packed up the family and moved to 'the country' – in this case, a 157-acre old dairy farm in northern Michigan – he was six years old. "My dad was a floor trader and investment advisor but my parents always wanted to try farming," Jimmy recalled. "So at age seventeen, I decided to pitch in and help."

"I plowed up a 10-acre hay field and planted vegetables. But to be honest, in the beginning, I was better at growing weeds (laughing). We started with a roadside stand and eggs were $1/doz. – eventually, I added some of my produce."

To survive they became a 'value-added farm.' Jimmy's mother Sharon began canning the excess vegetables, animals joined the farm and they began serving luncheons – evolving into an agritourism experience. Now, there are vegetables available the year-round, lunches served and wine tastings seven days a week, wine dinners and barn dances.

"As long as I can remember my mom was a home winemaker," Jimmy said. "Right in the center of the property is an elevation we called Sunset Hill because you can see beautiful sunsets on Lake Michigan from the top. I could see one day growing grapevines on that beautiful southern slope but didn't relish the thought of having to clear of all those trees. But the vision never faded."

Then Jim and Kim Palmer came on the scene as partners in the winery venture, which provided the necessary nudge to get the project moving forward. The hill was cleared and over three acres of vines were planted beginning in the spring of 2009 – four more acres will be added next year.

As the vineyard fruit becomes available, Harbor Springs Winery will be offering estate grown wines. In the meantime, there is an ample supply of quality fruit in the area and the winery is growing rapidly. Currently, there are thirteen wines and ciders available.

Interview with Jimmy Spencer:

You said your mother was a winemaker but was the vision for a winery there a long time?

Jimmy: I stared at that hill for years and thought 'one day I'm gonna grow grapes there but the hill was covered with trees, so my vision was a bit blurred (laughing). A winery was just another added dimension to Pond Hill Farm. I thought it would be perfect. Occasionally, I'd take the chainsaw up there and cut a few trees as needed but the big break came when I spotted a timber harvesting crew up the road one day. Normally they wouldn't come in for just a 5-acre site. All the pieces came together quickly – the hill was cleared and the vineyard/winery vision became much clearer.

Was the timber used to build your tasting room?

Jimmy: Some of the lumber was used for the store, the café and the tasting room walls and bar tops. All the buildings here were built with trees from the property – it all gets used on various projects eventually.

What was the reason for using Harbor Springs in your winery name?

Jimmy: We kicked around a lot of different names, like Pond Hill Winery and Tunnel of Trees Winery. But ultimately, everyone that comes into this area of Michigan can identify with Harbor Springs. It's a destination – the community, the resort environment and the water. We're proud of the town we live in and we think the name speaks to a larger customer base.

Here's my interpretation of your label: 'looking out open barn doors at a moon over the vineyards.' How close am I?

Jimmy: You would be correct. My wife, Marci, designed it. That shutter design is used on our livestock barn, inside the café and also in the tasting room.

So does Marci do the label design for the wines as well?

Jimmy: Marci works with a local artist who does the actual artwork and then she handles the graphic design. So I would call it a collaborative effort.

Where do the names Regatta Red and Tunnel Vision Cider come from?

Jimmy: The Regatta Red is named after the Ugotta Regatta on Little Traverse Bay, which is held right after the Chicago to Mackinaw boat race. Regatta weekend in Harbor Springs is a huge event for the town. Tunnel Vision Cider is named after the tunnel of trees that line M-119, which is a beautiful windy road that follows the shoreline and takes you right to Harbor Springs Winery and Pond Hill Farm. It does go further but we'd prefer you stop in and see us.

Where does the majority of your customer base come from?

Jimmy: Because we offer such a wide variety of activities and are family oriented, we're drawing many of the vacationers, both summer and winter, from literally everywhere. It's a diverse group and not uncommon to see license plates in the parking lot from any of the 50 states.

One of the big wine events in Harbor Springs is the Waterfront Wine Festival. Tell us about that.

Jimmy: It's an annual event put on by the Chamber of Commerce, which has multiple wine and food vendors, local artists and live music. I think it's a wonderful way for people to get a taste of northern Michigan. We look forward to pouring wine there every year.

Now tell us about the magic cork trick?

Jimmy: Our tasting room manager has a couple tricks he does with corks. But you have to try a few tastings before he'll divulge any secrets (laughing).

How would you describe the personality of your winery?

Jimmy: We love the homey non-intimidating atmosphere at the winery and the whole farm. I'd call it earthy and organic. I would say to expect a friendly atmosphere in natural surroundings.

Describe your mother, your wife and yourself using wine terms.

Jimmy: My mother is still very active here and everyone sees her as the heart of the business so she's a red that's aging well. If there were such a thing as 'royal wine' it would be her. My wife is the fresh wonderful white wine – a great mother, companion and friend…she's the pairing that goes with everything. I'm a young red wine that needs a little more time to age but hopefully getting better with time – definitely a work in progress (laughing).

A great variety for the wine rack – thanks Jimmy.

HEAVENLY VINEYARDS
Sometimes It's Meant To Be

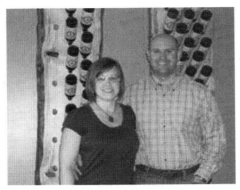

Ray Kroc, the founder of the McDonalds franchise, once said 'the two most important requirements for success are: first, being at the right place at the right time, and second, doing something about it.' Sandy and Aaron Sedine were and did. They had spotted a plot of land in Mecosta County just four miles east of U.S. 131. The last thing on their mind was a winery. But going from a dream place of property to making homemade wine to building Heavenly Vineyards wasn't a dream – it was just meant to be.

They were high school sweethearts from Coopersville (just west of Grand Rapids) and both attended Grand Valley University, with Sandy becoming a teacher and Aaron going into the family business with a mechanical engineering degree. Shortly after graduation, they got married and a wedding present became the spark to start a winery.

"It's strange to think a beer-making kit started it all," chuckled Aaron. "The kit made three moves to new homes before I finally said 'we either try this or throw it out.' That led to a wine kit and making fruit wines. Our first attempt was Concord, blueberry and cherry wines – nasty stuff, very high in alcohol and way past cordial, right to brandy."

Their winemaking improved dramatically. With encouragement from family and friends, the need to move the operation out of the house, purchasing the right land, the licensing process and the creation of Heavenly Vineyards all happened within two years.

"Aaron puts a lot of time in at his company and I teach school, so this is something the family can do together," Sandy said. "It keeps me busy picking and processing fruit in the summer and Aaron busy making wines in the winter."

The doors of Heavenly Vineyards opened and the Sedine's began sharing their wines with the world in April 2012.

Interview with Sandy and Aaron Sedine:

Your location is a bit off the traditional winery trails. How did you end up in Morley, Michigan?

Sandy: We looked at the property many years ago and were very interested in buying. We walked down into the woods by the creek and it was so peaceful and serene – I said to Aaron 'this is heavenly.' But the deal fell through, so we walked away. Eventually, we purchased that same property and the winery name was perfect – Heavenly Vineyards.

Aaron: We both loved it here, so I came to check again on its availability and this time the owner, who now lives in a nursing home, was three weeks from losing it to back taxes. I made him an offer and bought it within days. All the pieces fell in place very quickly and we started plans for the winery immediately – right place, right time.

The process to get a winery open can be tedious, with all the ordinances and regulations. Were there any major obstacles?

Sandy: No, other than the multiple hoops you have to jump through and the fact that the township had to create a bunch of new ordinances because we are the first and only winery around here.

Aaron: There was a run-down double-wide and dilapidated garage on the property and when the state inspector came, she was scratching her head, wondering 'this is gonna be a winery?' But I salvaged the garage for storage, tore everything else down and built the winery from scratch, so the next time she came to inspect, we got much more favorable looks (laughing).

Your labels feature a majestic tree. Is the tree significant and who designed it?

Sandy: I designed it – I have a graphic arts degree. Aaron has the business background, so he handles that part of the operation. He's the money/labor hunter and I'm the creative gatherer (laughing). The tree is a symbolic representation of the fantastic wooded area we're surrounded by, which was a big part of why we moved here.

The names of your wines are very creative, so I'm assuming that falls under the duties of the creative gatherer...

Sandy: Yes, most of the time it does. We do pick almost all of the fruit right here in Michigan – cherries, blackberries, blueberries, rhubarb, etc. which is stated on the label. I named our Pinot Noir red Capricious because that grape is sometimes hard to grow and VCR came from our homemade wine days. We didn't label the bottles back then, so we just put identifying initials on the cork – Vieux Chateau du Roi, VCR or Gewerztraminer is Big G.

Aaron: We've got an Uncle Jack who really got into that original high-octane black cherry wine. So we still make a 'milder' version of black cherry specialty wine, which we call Black Jack in his honor – but these batches are only 17% alcohol.

You are also attempting to grow your own grapes. How is that project coming along?

Aaron: So far, so good – they are about two years away from really producing quality grapes. At this time, rather than buy bulk juice, we prefer to press and process the whole grapes ourselves.

Sandy: This year we got the grapes from the Allegan area and are very pleased with the quality. And as I said, we try to gather as much fruit locally as possible.

Being only a few miles from U.S. 131 is a big plus but you're still an island unto yourself. How are you handling that challenge?

Sandy: Marketing is still our biggest problem. We're still working hard to get the wine tasters here. This year we'll be joining the West Michigan Wine and Beer Trail. And we're looking forward to having signage out on both north and southbound U.S. 131 near the Morley exits and on M-46.

You have a nice wine selection. How did you decide which wines to try?

Sandy: First we went with what we had already made that received a thumbs up from family and friends. We also used that system to eliminate some (laughing). But we also thought about what was different. For instance, we made a lemon wine and it sold out within a few months – so that's a keeper. We want to offer a good variety and still maintain high quality.

Aaron: We're also willing to think outside the box to distinguish ourselves from everyone else. I made a pineapple wine and we sent out emails to our customers to have them come in a try it and give us feedback. It got a good response as well. We want to make wines you can't buy at Meijer.

So, overall, this hobby turned business was a good idea?

Sandy: Originally, it was something that would keep me busy in the summer and I could have my kids around and involved. It's not something we need to do but rather something we both enjoy and want to do.

Aaron: It's such a pleasure to be able to share this experience with others. We've both enjoyed meeting the people and have made some great friends. Not everyone wants to go all the way up north to enjoy good wine or have to battle 50 to 100 others in the tasting rooms. Heavenly Vineyards offers a quality intimate experience with a personal touch.

So you don't have to go THAT far to taste some different wines, have a great time and make a new friend. Thanks guys.

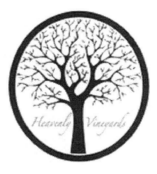

See Heavenly Vineyards ad on page 408.

**To do list: buy wine, open wine, pour wine, drink wine.
REPEAT**

LEFT FOOT CHARLEY WINERY
Relax With Both Feet Up

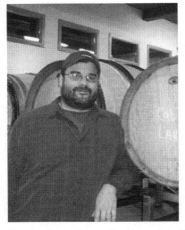

First, Left Foot Charley is really Bryan Ulbrich. Second, you know there's a story behind that – more, later. Third, it's hard to believe you can kick back and enjoy a nice glass of wine while surrounded by the ambiance of the former Northern Michigan Asylum in Traverse City. Believe it!

"Americans can finally relax," says winemaker and proprietor Bryan Ulbrich. "People used to always say 'let's go out for a beer or a drink' – they rarely said 'let's go out for a glass of wine' – well, that's finally changing. We want to take the wine tasting experience to the next level and make it an everyday experience."

Originally from suburban Chicago, Ulbrich used to visit the Traverse City area spending summer vacations with his grandparents. After going off to college, first in Indiana then Arizona, Bryan returned in 1995 and decided he didn't want to leave.

Having learned the rudimentary workings of the business while employed at a winery out west, he and his soon to be bride Jennifer, realized northern Michigan was the place to settle. After answering a "winery help needed" ad from the newspaper,

Ulbrich began an "all-encompassing" apprenticeship with Peninsula Cellars in 1996. "Dave Kroupa (vineyard owner) taught me how to fix things, build things and work the land. Lee Lutes (winemaker) taught me how to dress, wear comfortable shoes, ferment grapes and sell wine (laughing)."

After Lutes moved on to Black Star Farms, Ulbrich continued making award-winning wines at Peninsula Cellars until he took the leap and produced his own vintage in 2004. Left Foot Charley became a reality in 2006 and is located in what is now known as The Village at Grand Traverse Commons.

Interview with Bryan Ulbrich:

Ok, let's get it out of the way…you are Left Foot Charley – explanation please.

Bryan: Yes, I am Left Foot Charley but the origins are somewhat vague. My mother always liked Charles Schultz, so, in honor of Charlie Brown, I was tagged with the nickname at an early age. But recently we've discovered it might have also been a WWII era substitute phrase for swearing. My grandfather was a WWII vet but so far, no one in the family is confessing, so we're still investigating (laughing).

You got started just prior to a huge expansion in the Michigan wine industry. What was it like before the explosion in winery numbers?

Bryan: I think there were only three wineries on Old Mission Peninsula and maybe a half dozen on Leelanau. But in the late 1990's and early 2000's, there was a large influx of investment money and, although some have changed hands now, to my knowledge none of them have gone under. I used to go to the Michigan Annual Meetings and knew everyone there. Now, you really need a nametag.

What are the biggest differences you see in starting a winery back then and now?

Bryan: There is a radical difference in how the money is invested – especially in the areas of planting, the vine structure and preparing the soils. The amount spent on the winery itself is staggering as well. It's not the sexy image of the old man tilling the hillside with his horse anymore. To get into the international wine conversation, we need modern tools and that is very expensive. Just look at the crush pad at Chateau Grand Traverse – its on par with anything in the world. I look at our facility and just shake my head at how far we've come.

Has this new technology had an effect on the quality of Michigan wines?

Bryan: Yes, a dramatic improvement. With new techniques, better equipment, higher quality personnel and higher quality fruit, Michigan is producing great tasting wines that have changed the perception in the entire wine industry. Out on the road, selling wine, it's gone from 'your wine sucks' to 'that's not bad' to 'we want to feature your wine!'

So, it's a tough road out there selling Michigan wine…

Bryan: In the early days, it was brutal. But Michigan wineries have worked hard to not only improve the quality of wines we produce but to work on all those cynics and convert them to customers. It's so nice when someone calls today and NEEDS ten cases right now and you can say 'I'm sorry – I'm all out but I can get one case out of my library or I can put you on the list for next year's vintage.' That makes this business a lot more fun.

You don't grow your own grapes but rather get them from local vineyards. How does that work?

Bryan: Our model is more expensive than if we just bought the juice. We treat the growers better than a market-based model. Their take is based on the bottle price rather than sugar levels or chemistry – they're paid on historical quality. Its more than the money, they want a reputation for producing high quality grapes, which in turn makes a better and higher priced wine. It has worked very well for both sides and quite frankly couldn't be done without cooperation and a good working relationship.

When did you get the vision for Left Foot Charley?

Bryan: It started with offering to salvage a portion of a new vineyard owner's crop. That turned into 200 bottles of Riesling, which then evolved into working with a couple of custom clients to build a custom crushing facility using a co-op type model for producing wine. We took the leap and settled on trying to build a winery in town rather than on one of the traditional peninsula wine trails.

And so the Village as a location became a reality…

Bryan: The renovation of this whole facility has been fantastic and we believe in the Village concept. I like old buildings and the whole re-purposing idea. Our winery is located in the Asylum's laundry building. I showed my wife the blown out windows and the 20 years of dirt and bird droppings and to her credit, she just said 'Whatever, if you believe in it.' So, I took all of our savings (laughing) and we're still here.

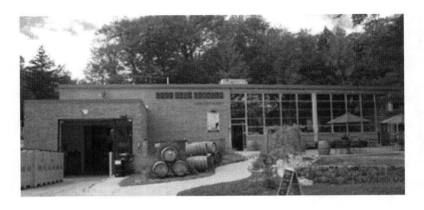

How does your operation differ from the traditional winery tasting rooms?

Bryan: The traditional model is based on a 30-minute turnover – taste the wine, buy the wine, move on. We expect our customer to stay longer, that's why we put in stools and tables. We cater to the locals as well as the tourist. It's patterned after a more European model – wine by the glass, a little bit of food - and it works. Hard ciders have been a huge addition to our tasting room. It adds to the atmosphere, the image of the winery and softens the wine edge.

You have reasonably priced wines but is it just the quality that raises the price?

Bryan: In reality, for a small winery, it's the people – the number of hands - look at a bottle of wine and think of the number of hands that have worked to make it possible. That is a rather simplistic explanation but we can mechanize the process and make cheaper wine. Without those hands, it would be mostly machinery. It's the human touch that adds the expense but isn't wine worth it?

Indeed it is, thanks Bryan.

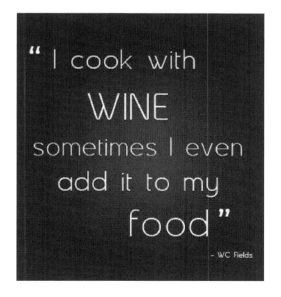

NORTHERN NATURAL WINERY
Wine For The Health of It

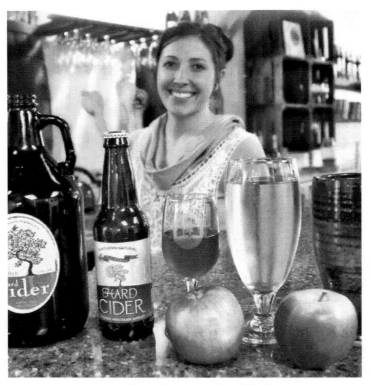

Northern Natural – Jen Mackey

Northern Natural Organics is a small family farming operation committed to growing certified organic fruits. Northern Natural Winery is committed to making great tasting wines and ciders. The two have created a natural pairing.

Dennis Mackey and his partners established Northern Natural Organics in 1997, which is an organic juice production facility supporting eight certified organic family fruit farms in Michigan. In 2009, he crafted his first batch of traditional hard cider.

It was his passion for growing quality fruits that sparked a conversation with winemaker Shawn Walters and the ultimate creation of a winery featuring organic fruits. Northern Natural Winery opened in 2009 with eight ciders on draft. They've grown rapidly and now have a product list with thirteen wines and five hard ciders.

Still a family operation, Dennis concentrates on the farming and juice production, son Kyle handles the cider production and cooking duties and daughter-in-law Jen Mackey is the Director and Sales Manager of the winery and Northern Natural Organics.

Although wine drinkers loved the fruit wines at the tasting room in Benzonia, it quickly became apparent there was a need for more, so traditional varietals and blends were added. The entire tasting room operation was moved to Front Street in downtown Traverse City in 2013.

One very popular item is their hard cider. "We do have some people who are attracted to our wines because of our fruit growing process," Jen said. " But what's most exciting is hearing people who just love our award-winning hard ciders and wines because they come from locally grown vineyards and orchards."

We have it on good authority, you can't make a bad choice from the diverse line of organic foods paired with the wines and ciders they're offering.

Interview with Jen Mackey:

As a family owned and operated winery, you can't avoid business at the dinner table. How do those dynamics work?

Jen: Oh, we're always in total agreement on everything (laughing). Actually, one of our customers, who also is part of a family owned business put it best...you don't always see eye to eye but you can't operate without each other, so there's a respect for everyone involved. Ultimately, we have the same goal, which is for the business to succeed.

How would you define 'organic?'

Jen: Our organic practices are under the Global Alliance Certification – all natural fertilizers, no pesticides and mineralization of the soil without using chemical additives.

There is a lot of documentation about organic being healthier but that also means, for the most part, more expensive. Is that still the case?

Jen: When I first started, yes, that was true. Some customers would pass up 'organic' based on product price points. Today, we're getting as many, if not more, who understand and accept the reasons for 'organic' and seek us out. Prices are very competitive and even comparable now.

But just to clarify – your wines aren't 100% organic?

Jen: The wines aren't certified organic but when made with our fruit – it's made with 100% certified organic fruit. Our winemaker grows sustainable wine grapes, which are not organic, for use in some of our varietal and blended wines.

So, is that why you don't mention organic in your slogan, which is 'Locally Owned – Locally Grown'?

Jen: Yes – even though the majority of the fruit we use is organic we also support other farms that are not certified but practice similar growing techniques.

I've read about the health benefits of drinking wine (in moderation), so I'm assuming wine made with 100% organic fruit is even more beneficial. Do your customers think that as well?

Jen: The public's awareness regarding the benefits of organic fruit is as close to 'taken for granted' as it will ever be…a customer may ask 'how' but the 'why' is rarely an issue.

Speaking of rare, I understand you make something called 'Iced Apple Cider' and it is very hard to find.

Jen: We were originally one of two wineries that produced Iced Apple Cider in 2009 – so it is pretty rare. It takes over 42 lbs. of apples for one bottle and has a balanced sweetness from start to finish.

Who created the Rockin Robin brand?

Jen: That was Kyle's sister Alison, who is a graphics designer. It's based on the robin being Michigan's state bird. All the fruit in that brand is grown on our farm.

The new tasting room in Traverse City has definite 'orchard' highlights. Tell us about your decorations.

Jen: We brought in some 50-year-old apple and cherry wood to make tables, benches and bar tops for the tasting house. It's decorated with wine barrels, apple crates and wheels from an old juice line. You're in the city but you can feel the farm orchard atmosphere.

Your husband Kyle graduated from the Great Lakes Culinary Institute. What is his specialty and does he do the cooking at home?

Jen: Not only does he cook at home but he's the chef out at the production facility as well. Pizza is his specialty and he incorporated seasonal local organic produce for toppings.

What wine fits your father-in-law's personality and pick yours as well.

Jen: That's tough because he likes sweet wines and I prefer a drier wine. I'll go with the Rockin Robin Strawberry Wine for his personality type and I'm going with the crisp and refreshing Cherry Lemongrass Hard Cider.

I'll take all the extra health benefits I can get – more organic please – thanks Jen

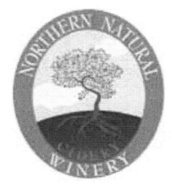

See Northern Natural's ad on page 411.

NORTHEAST

MODERN CRAFT..151
ROSE VALLEY..156
STONEY ACRES..162
THUNDER BAY...167
VALLEY MIST...172

MODERN CRAFT WINERY
The First Stop On The Sunrise Side
Wine & Hops Trail

Skip the mimosa – close your eyes – you're sipping a glass of grapefruit blush and can hear the waves lapping at the shore of Lake Huron – you're on the patio of Modern Craft Winery in Au Gres.

One of Michigan's newest fast-track wineries, Modern Craft has only been open since November 2011 but they already have a large selection of wines to choose from. Just off U.S. 23, the tasting room is literally within sight of Saginaw Bay.

One of the owners, Jeff Czymbor, was a true neophyte when it came to wine making. But the entrepreneurial spirit was there from an early age. His first business was started while he was still a high school student in St. Charles, MI. "My neighbor, who was in his 90's at the time, owned a building in Saginaw that used to be a printing shop. I wasn't very scholarly (laughing), so he helped me get everything into shape. It became Printing Edge Publishing and the rest is history, as they say."

Fast-forward thirty years and Jeff's business is so successful, he goes into semi-retirement, moves to Au Gres in 2009 and another elderly neighbor comes into the picture. This one was a winemaking hobbyist. "He couldn't move the barrels around anymore, so I volunteered. Along the way, he became a mentor and pretty soon, all available space in my house was filled with wine barrels."
You can only do so much fishing and relaxing...so eventually the itch to start something new needed to be scratched, and Modern Craft Winery was born.

Interview with Jeff Czymbor:

The leap from homemade wines to licensed winery is a big leap. Did you just have an insane moment?

Jeff: Most definitely (laughing). My wife, Jennifer, and I started going to a neighborhood Tuesday gathering, which became known as Narnia night – friends bringing a dish to pass, kids playing and adults drinking wine in April 2011. I soon discovered that Tom Nixon also had a passion for making wine. Two weeks later, Narnia was at my house and we started the licensing process that night. By November, ironically 11-11-11, Modern Craft Winery was a reality. And yes, we probably had a little too much wine back in April.

How did the name Modern Craft come about?

Jeff: We started the licensing process online and modern technology took over – it disappeared off the computer screen and was inadvertently submitted, which started the clock ticking to complete the process or you have to start over from scratch. We had a list of potential winery names but the first one we applied for said Modern Craft because we weren't going to make our wines the traditional way. We've patented our winemaking processes, i.e. a modern craft. That technological mistake with the computer probably saved us hours and hours of hassling over a name.

Was the winery logo submitted at the same time?

Jeff: No, the logo has evolved several times. The label approval process is always ongoing but I guess we're basically satisfied with the current one…until another logo comes up that we like better (laughing).

Did you look to model your winery/business plan after an existing operation or go your own way?

Jeff: That was an interesting process. I've always been inspired by my father's work ethic. He retired from the Navy and went to work and eventually retired from GM. But we didn't want to work harder than the competition; we wanted to do it smarter. So, yes, in that sense, we were thinking outside the box from the very beginning. My dad still works too hard but at least it's for us now.

Your wine list has grown rapidly – tell us about selecting a wine that makes it to the tasting room.

Jeff: Well, for people who knew absolutely nothing about the wine industry, we've come up with some good wines that our customers love. Our first step was eliminating the ones our wives thought tasted terrible. It truly was a trial and error situation in the beginning but that also helped us not get trapped into making the traditional wine making mistakes. We quickly moved into processing techniques that are proprietary and make our wines taste great.

When you bottle your wine, is there a closure preference?

Jeff: We use bar tops, synthetic and real cork depending on the type of wine we're bottling and what closure we think will work best. As long as it makes a good seal and doesn't affect the taste, I don't think it really matters.

What was the best advice you got starting this new venture into the wine business?

Jeff: Assuming you are starting with a high quality product, which I think we have, the best advice regarding the success or failure of the winery was understanding the importance of the number of people you can get through the doors of your tasting room. It may sound over simplified but a great tasting wine doesn't sell unless you get people to try it.

What was the biggest obstacle to overcome in attracting people to your tasting room?

Jeff: We have a beautiful aesthetic building but we're five miles off of U.S. 23, which is the main corridor to northeast Michigan and runs right through Au Gres. So getting the proper signs in the optimal locations was critical. Our guest logbooks have shown a large percentage of customers are from out of state. Knowing that now, we will adjust our marketing to promote that trend.

You must get a big smile on your face when you see a bus pull up to the tasting room…what gives you the most satisfaction in starting your winery?

Jeff: Build it and they will come (laughing) and thank goodness they are!

And now you've developed the Sunrise Side Wine & Hops Trail. Tell us about that.

Jeff: For being as new as it is, we are very pleased with the positive results. The members work well together and send each other business. We like to think of it as an invitation into our home. It's less business-driven and more family/people oriented. It's a beautiful drive up the sunrise side.

It certainly is, thanks Jeff.

ROSE VALLEY WINERY
The Days Of Wine And Roses

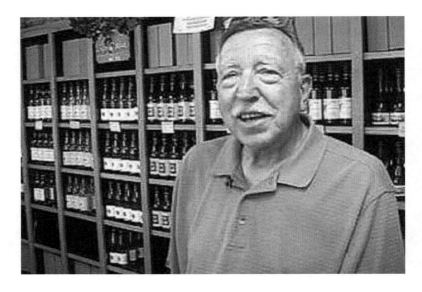

There are few roses but there is plenty of good wine just a few blocks from of the main intersection in the small town of Rose City in Ogemaw County. Adam Kolodziejski, the owner of the Rose Valley Winery, is the magician behind taking ordinary grapes and making extraordinary wines.

The son of a Polish immigrant, Adam grew up just nineteen miles east of the winery in Hale, Michigan. It is there on the old homestead farm, which he now calls Hunting Hawk Vineyard, where he planted nearly thirty varieties of grapes. Many of the vines are native to Michigan but he also brought in a multitude of cold-hardy grapes that have thrived under his care.

From humble beginnings, Adam quickly understood the value of stretching the dollar. "I learned you can make three cups of tea from one tea bag if it's properly cared for," he chuckled. When he discovered he was not ready for college yet, he joined the Merchant Marines. Several years later, he discovered the mail hadn't caught up to him in quite a while (which included a few military induction notices) and there was a U.S. Marshal waiting on the docks in Baltimore accusing him of dodging the draft. Some fast talking was followed by a 4-year stint in the Navy.

The GI Bill helped him get a teaching certificate from CMU but after one year in the classroom – 'that was enough for me' – he worked in industry and eventually started his own metal manufacturing company.

Years later, Adam won first prize in a contest – either $25,000 in gold pesos or a plot of land at a retirement resort in Mexico. Being a farmer's son, he took the land. As age sixty approached, he thought he'd check it out. "It quickly became apparent why my neighbors were all drinking tequila at the Cantina by mid-morning," he recalled. "Everyone, including me, was bored silly. But one of the non-curriculum skills I learned in college was making wine. So, I packed up, flew home, started planting vines and making plans to build a winery. I guess retirement wasn't in my genetic pool."

He broke ground in 2004 and opened Rose Valley Winery in 2006.

Interview with Adam Kolodziejski:

How did you decide on your winery name?

Adam: It's a nice catchy name...it's in Rose City but there are some restrictions on using names of actual geographic places. The city welcomed me in with my manufacturing business and I wanted to show my appreciation and support by giving at least partial identity to them. I've been here for seven years and I still get a few locals in who say 'I didn't know there was a winery just down the street!' I just smile and tell'em 'you gotta get out more.'

You also identified some rivers and lakes in the area when naming your wines.

Adam: Yes, like our Rifle River Red and Lake Ambrose White. We also sold Clear Lake White for a couple years but the Feds made us stop because Clear Lake is a viticulture area in California. It seems I can only get away with things for a short time before the law catches up with me (laughing).

What is your opinion on box wines?

Adam: My experience with box wines is limited. I bought a box of wine once and put it in the refrigerator. I drank and drank and drank from that darn box and it seemed like it took two years to finish it. So I decided to sell my wine by the bottle because I want my customers to come back eventually (laughing).

How did you decide on the wines you make?

Adam: Sometimes it's 'I want to try this' and other times it's arguing with Steve (the winemaker). Our goal is to make very traditional wines and make them well, which does limit us on the wild and crazy things you can do. For instance, our Red Table

Wine I think is well made and doesn't need to be 'tickled up' with subtle nuances to make it adventuresome. It stands on its own and we hope our customers appreciate that. There is a market for what I call 'pop' wines for $4 a bottle but we're trying to stick with a conventional wine list and not venture too far.

Usually, it's the bigger wineries that can afford to market a loss leader or rock bottom priced wine. How do you price your wines?

Adam: In our case, it's a labor of love because we're not getting rich. But we've also chosen to stay small. Our cost, what the market will bear, sweat equity and profit margin are all factors. One day we'll figure out how to make some money (laughing).

What have you found to be the most satisfying part of owning a winery?

Adam: When all those women come in on a Saturday and they want to meet and give the winemaker a hug. I give'em all a big hug and sometimes they come back for seconds – no thirds though because my wife draws the line. Really, I do enjoy interacting with the customers. We get a lot of first-time visitors who've never been to a winery. So we give them a tour and take the time to educate them on how to drink wine. I also get a lot of satisfaction from growing and making wine from a new style grape, the cold-hardy varieties that were developed specifically for northern climates.

How have they done at your vineyard?

Adam: They have done very well. They don't freeze out in the winter and bud out late in the spring, which avoids the late spring frost and it's generally more disease resistant than European vinifera. We can harvest our grapes by Labor Day weekend or if we consult our weather crystal ball and if we see a mild fall in the forecast, some years it's late October before we're taking in the last of the harvest. It gives Michigan winemakers a lot of latitude.

To get specific, the sugar content of grapes is measured in 'brix.' What are normal sugar levels in Michigan grapes compared to California grapes?

Adam: Many times a Michigan grape never gets the weather to reach its peak or ideal level, which would be somewhere around 21-22 brix. California grape sugar levels are around the mid-20's. But they have the opposite problem – they struggle to keep the grapes from over-ripening. Once a grape gets too ripe, the acid levels drop dramatically and the flavors are sweet but bland – no essence left that gives wine that special/interesting taste. The sugar/acid balance is key to making good wine and the hybrid grapes give Michigan winemakers the opportunity to fine-tune that balance.

In your opinion, what makes Rose Valley Winery unique?

Adam: There is an old saying: 'if you're going to make wine – make wine; if you're going to grow grapes – grow grapes…don't do both.' But I'm Polish, so here I am doing both. I also point out on the tours that I flunked Chemistry in school (laughing). We want our guests to experience a warm friendly atmosphere – to enjoy our traditional but unique wines. Our staff works hard to put smiles on their faces and hopefully, they leave with a desire to come visit us again.

Mission accomplished! I'm already looking forward to my next visit. Thanks Adam.

See the Rose Valley Winery ad on page 414.

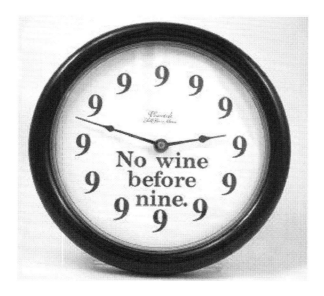

WINE AND CHOCOLATE
A MATCH MADE AT STONEY ACRES WINERY

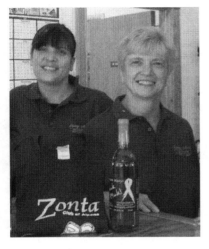

If you travel up the sunrise side of Michigan, as you're leaving Alpena just north of town, you may catch a whiff of chocolate. If your throat is a bit parched, the lure of good fruit wines will pull you right to the door of Jim and Helen Grochowski's Stoney Acres Winery. To most, it's a tough combination to resist and you won't be disappointed.

Just when the notion of starting a winery came about seems to have become a family secret. "My dad is the winemaker but when that seed of turning a hobby into a business was planted, he's not saying," said daughter and business manager Amy Gagnon.

Jim learned to make wine the 'old school' way from his grandparents in their basement with 10-gallon crocks. "I can still remember those fermenting smells coming from under the basement stairwell," laughed Amy. "It always stays with you." Before long, that space under the stairs couldn't hold all the crocks.

Eventually, the basement was filling with 55-gallon barrels and Helen finally said 'enough.' Everything moved to Jim's 40 x 60 workshop out back in the early 1990's. Gradually, enough people told them 'this wine is really good – you should start marketing it to the public.'

They were officially licensed in 1999 and opened a tasting room in 2001. With grapes still scarce in the area, they turned to what they always liked and concentrated on other fruits that are prevalent in the Alpena area. It seems very appropriate that customers step up to the long tasting room bar Jim made out of fieldstones picked from the surrounding stone-laden acres.

Interview with Amy Gagnon:

Let's assume there are a lot of stones around…is that where the name came from?

Amy: You might say that. I had a horse when I was younger and had to dig fence postholes. I must have hit a couple thousand rocks, at least. We wanted to pick a unique name and had a long list of ideas. It was almost named Fall Creek Winery, which is a creek on my Grandparents property that empties into Thunder Bay. There's also a lot of swampland in the area but we didn't wanna go there (laughing). My dad used fieldstone for building foundations, retaining walls and the tasting room bar so the name choice really does fit our location.

Your label/logo is a picture of your parent's home. What's the history on that choice?

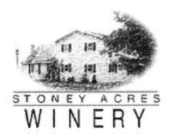

Amy: When the idea of developing the winery happened I was working for the local newspaper and doing a lot of graphics work. We took a picture of the house, changed the angle and turned it into line art – everyone loved it. Originally, the label said Stoney Acres Winery, Alpena, Michigan. But I began to think 'why state the obvious on a bottle of wine' so we just went with Stoney Acres.

Your selection concentrates primarily on non-grape fruit wines. Why?

Amy: Historically, my dad made wine from what he knew and grew and just a few grape varietals can survive up here in the northeast. But the other fruits we use in our wines are locally sourced – many of them have been with us from the very beginning. We use Knaebe's Munchy Crunchy apples from Roger City, blueberries from Tawas, cranberries from Cheboygan, raspberries from Ossineke and strawberries from AJ's in Lachine. At the time we started, it was risky. There were only a few other wineries in Michigan that had a selection made up of non-grape wines.

In general, do you find it easy to pick out what customers will like?

Amy: Usually, in three samples from the tasting room, I can tell what they'll like. But we do something very unique here – we make each variety of wine in various levels of sweetness. For example, we have a semi-dry and semi-sweet raspberry wine. In our Silver City White, we have a choice of dry, semi-dry and semi-sweet. We've found that in many cases, a couple will come in and like the same variety but two different levels of sweetness.

Stoney Acres also provides supplies and ingredients for the 'winemaking hobbyist' and now, (practically every woman's dream) chocolate to go with the wine. How did that start?

Amy: My parents started selling the supplies & ingredients out of the house before they opened the winery. Our winery is very dependant on tourism and someone told us about a boutique winery in California that served chocolate with their raspberry wine. So, we went out and researched all kinds of chocolate – a lot of chocolates (laughing). We eventually hired a chocolatier who made our gourmet truffles. She has since moved on but taught us her recipe before leaving and we have added chocolate bars, chocolate peanut brittle and a very decadent triple chocolate drizzle caramel corn.

When someone comes in with the idea of making wine in their home, what is a good piece of advice to start with?

Amy: Start keeping a journal, at the very beginning. Everything you do – write it down. When you run into a problem, which everyone does at sometime, there is no way to track your progress if there isn't proper documentation. We can't advise you on a problem if we don't know what you've done. Sometimes, it can be 'three strikes, you're out' or 'the third time's the charm.'

What is the most common question you get from customers in the tasting room?

Amy: I would say it's probably 'what wine do I serve with this food.' We are constantly educating our customers on how wine flavors change with what you're eating. Sometimes they buy a wine after trying it in the tasting room, take it home and serve it with a certain food and then its 'wow, that doesn't taste good.' Don't assume it must be a bad bottle of wine. Give wine a chance to be the wonderful tasting experience it's supposed to be.

Let's finish the experience with three wines that best describes you and your parents.

Amy: My mom would be our new black raspberry wine Midnight Romance – she once said she wanted the wine to speak raspberry (meaning to be more full bodied) but I told her if the berries were speaking to her, she'd had too much to drink (laughing). My dad is the Silver City Red, deep and dry. Me, I'm our Think Pink Wine, which is an exotic fruit flavored white zinfandel. From personal experience, I know how important breast cancer awareness is for women. Those are three great Stoney Acres wines.

With a little chocolate chaser, thanks Amy.

THUNDER BAY WINERY
Where Hard Work Is Paying Off

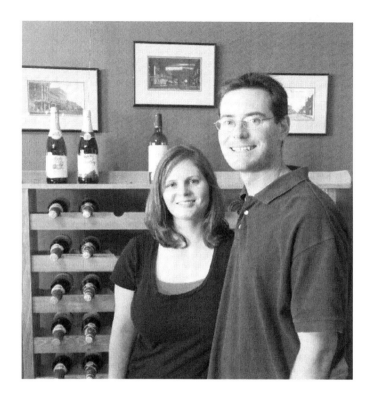

Even the locals are surprised when they find out grapes are grown and wine is being made in Alpena, Michigan. They shouldn't be surprised for several reasons.

Geographically, Alpena and Thunder Bay are near the 45th parallel, as is the Thunder Bay Winery owned by Jeremy and Janis Sahr. The winery is located in the historic Center Building in the heart of downtown Alpena and the owners are winning the hearts of wine drinkers with good wine as the number of visitors continues to increase.

If you follow the 45th parallel around the globe, one quickly discovers it runs through the premier wine country of the world – Bordeaux, France; Piedmont, Italy, Willamette, Oregon, Leelanau peninsula, Michigan and yes, Thunder Bay in Alpena. County.

Having a desire to make wine from an early age seems a bit strange considering Jeremy's background. "I wasn't raised on a farm nor is there any farming in our immediate family," he said. "I started making wine in a friend's closet, primarily because I didn't want my parents to find out (laughing) but in college I also found myself reading viticulture books in Psychology class."

He and Janis met while working at the Olive Garden restaurant in Saginaw. After they married, they headed up the sunrise side of the state in pursuit of Jeremy's dream of growing grapes and starting a winery. "It was truly blind faith," he recalled. "We both took jobs in a restaurant in Alpena until Janis finished her teaching degree. With a vineyard in mind, we purchased a home and 10-acres on an old strawberry farm and started planting vines the next spring."

That land is just a tick off the 45th parallel and has become the Thunder Bay Vineyards, established in 2005. The dream was complete when the Thunder Bay Winery opened its doors in 2012.

Interview with Jeremy Sahr:

I must say, most people don't think of Alpena when 'wine country' is mentioned. So, why Alpena?

Jeremy: Ironically, I came up here on a bike trip right out of high school and rode down the same road we live on now. I can remember thinking the rolling hills looked just like wine country – without the vines. Janis has relatives up here and we both just fell in love with the area. We did look at the Traverse City area but it was too crowded and expensive for us. We jumped in with both feet – it probably would have been easier had we taken it in steps (laughing) but we have no regrets.

If it weren't for the surrounding buildings, you could see Thunder Bay from here. Is that what inspired the winery name?

Jeremy: We like the maritime theme and we liked the idea of keeping a local connection. Even though there are other businesses with Thunder Bay in their name, it still sounded nice and everyone has responded positively to the choice.

With Alpena being a Great Lakes port, you've also carried the maritime theme on your labels.

Jeremy: Yes, our specialty wines reflect local landmarks like Starlight Beach and Sugar Island. We've got plans to include some of the more famous shipwrecks and lighthouses in the area. Janis and I both appreciate the history up here and we are using a 1913 map of Thunder Bay for our winery logo and on the labels as well.

What have you found to be the most difficult part of owning a winery?

Jeremy: The actual making of the wine is one of the easiest – but growing the grapes, good quality grapes, is much more difficult. Time management is another issue with owning a business because, obviously, you have to take the time to market and sell the wine to be successful.

Are you angling to make it an 'Estate' winery?

Jeremy: We have three acres planted with plenty of room to expand. Time will tell. About 40% of our wines come from our own vineyard grapes but all the rest are Michigan grown. We do outsource some blackberries from Washington and the cranberries come from a company that's right on the Wisconsin/Michigan border, so some of them might be Michigan cranberries (laughing). We've made a commitment to support local growers as much as possible.

It must be a challenge to even convince people that grapes can grow here. Do you encounter that disbelief much?

Jeremy: Yes, even from people who've lived here their whole lives and grow their own fruit! 'You grow grapes here?!' But that's also one of my greatest kicks – having them try a glass of our wine, made from grapes we've grown on our property and seeing a big smile on their face after saying 'this is really good.'

Your winery is actually located right in downtown Alpena. Has that created challenges?

Jeremy: We're actually on two floors – I spilled some wine the other day and it settled over in a different location. So, first that wasn't good and second, the floor obviously isn't level. It's an old building so regulating the heat is a big challenge. We've got a big picture window in front and we never thought about it steaming up in the winter (laughing). People always ask about where the wine comes from and we tell them it's made next door and they say 'ahah.' Then we show them and they say 'oh, you meant RIGHT next door.'

Just out of curiosity, when you're at a wine conference sitting around with other winemakers, what do you talk about?

Jeremy: We act just like a bunch of old farmers. We talk about the weather or the new grape variety on the horizon (substitute wheat, corn, sugar beets, etc.). Sometimes there's a discussion about a new growing technique someone is trying but for the most part, I think a wine drinker would find it very boring.

Do your wines reflect your personality?

Jeremy: Wow, this is like a weird job interview question – what tree would best describe you (laughing). I do want to make good quality traditional wines but I'm also not afraid to step outside the box and experiment. For instance, I'm making a wine from a North Dakota grape, which has an unbelievably intense flavor. It's different but I think people will love it. So, maybe that answers your question. Janis is the levelheaded person in the business and I'm the creative person. That sounds better than crazy doesn't it?

A winery in Alpena…I'd say crazy like a fox. Thanks Jeremy.

VALLEY MIST VINEYARDS
On The Edge of Wine Country

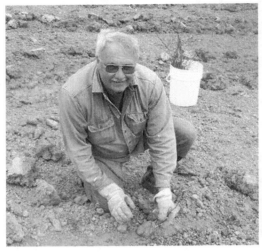

How does a beer and scotch drinker from Ypsilanti end up in Rose City making wine? Brad Moore's explanation makes sense – 'it was a home hobby that got out of control.'
His hobby was transformed into Valley Mist Vineyards and the winery lights burn late into the night to keep his wine on the shelves.

How do you recognize an avid home winemaker? The basement carpet is stained purple. Brad admits he loves making 'the stuff' but doesn't drink much wine and practically gave his away to anyone who wanted to try it. "Everyone kept telling me the wine was really good," Brad said. "But I thought they were just being nice."

He eventually grew tired of the southeast Michigan 'rat race' in the world of manufacturing and finance, which prompted a move to Rose City. His gardening green thumb inspired the idea to grow his own grapes and led to a trip across town to visit Adam Kolodziejski at the Rose Valley Winery.

"I mentioned to Adam I was thinking about planting a dozen or so vines," Brad recalled. "He asked me how much land I had and when I told him about three acres, he said 'if you plant it all in grapes, I'll buy all of it.' And 1,500 vines, 8 miles of wire and 600 trellis posts later, that's basically how the vineyard started."

After being downsized in his job of 35 years in 2009, Brad crunched the numbers and decided adding a winery to his vineyard was feasible. "Now I wish I would have lost my job years ago," he chuckled. "I actually come out and stand in my 401K each day."

In the first year of operation, he doubled his expectations and the business just kept growing. Valley Mist Vineyards is on the Sunrise Side Wine and Hops Trail and offers wines with 'unusual' names at reasonable prices – and they taste unusually good.

Interview with Brad Moore:

How did you come up with the name Valley Mist?

Brad: I was looking out my window one morning and the entire vineyard was shrouded in fog. You can see the mist just roll through the valleys here each fall.

Where does your juice/grapes come from and is the plan to become an estate winery?

Brad: We get plums, nectarines and apricots from Traverse City. The peaches come from a northern Michigan orchard and the Edelweiss grapes from Alpena. There is great 'co-opetition' in the wine industry and everyone tries to help whenever possible. As the yield from my own vineyard increases we will continue to use more and more estate grown grapes but I don't know if I'll ever be a 100% estate winery – time will tell.

Did you have a mentor?

Brad: Yes, Adam at Rose Valley has really been a reliable source of assistance and has mentored me along the way, especially when I began planting the vineyard. He has also allowed me to make use of his equipment as well. He's been a great help.

What sources of information and education did you use when starting your winery?

Brad: I just started reading everything I could find about making wine. The Internet is packed with websites about the whole industry. The actual process of making wine isn't difficult or "rocket science" – it's a pretty basic process with grapes or really any fruit you are using to make wine. MSU came out with two seminars just as I was getting started that also helped. One was for starting a winery – the other was for starting a vineyard. It was perfect timing for me. They had world-class speakers there and it was invaluable information.

Where did your creative wine names come from?

Brad: We sit around drinking beer, wine and scotch until the inspiration hits and we all agree on a name. Sometimes it takes a while (laughing). Lighting Bug Lemon Wine (aka Skeeter Pee) actually came from a recipe I got from a home winemaker's blog and no pun intended – it flies off the shelf. What can I say – the inspiration just flows (laughing).

You aren't far off M-55 but certainly are located in a non-traditional wine region. But you are thriving on 'uniqueness.'

Brad: Most definitely – we advertise and promote 'living on the edge.' We're not your typical winery – classic rock blasting in the background – not your traditional chamber music. I wouldn't say we cater to bikers but you do get a discount on wines if you show up on a Harley. There's a good chance you'll find wines here that you won't find anywhere else and there's a good chance if you show up here once, you'll definitely be back again.

Let me clarify myself – you're on the edge of your own wine region – thanks Brad.

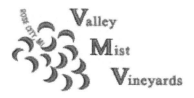

SOUTHWEST

BARODA FOUNDERS……………………………………...177
CASCADE……………………………………………………..184
CODY KRESTA………………………………………………..189
CONTESSA……………………………………………………196
DOMAINE BERRIEN…………………………………………201
FENN VALLEY…...……………………………………………208
GLASS CREEK………………………………………………215
GRAVITY……………………………………………………220
HICKORY CREEK……………………………………………226
HOMETOWN…………………………………………………...231
KARMA VISTA………………………………………………...236
LAWTON RIDGE……………………………………………242
ROBINETTES…………………………………………………248
ST. JULIEN……………………………………………………254
12 CORNERS…………………………………………………...261
WHITE PINE…………………………………………………267

If I ever go missing, I want my picture on a wine bottle instead of a milk carton. This way, my friends will know I'm missing.

BARODA FOUNDERS CELLAR
Oh Hell Yeah – He's Good

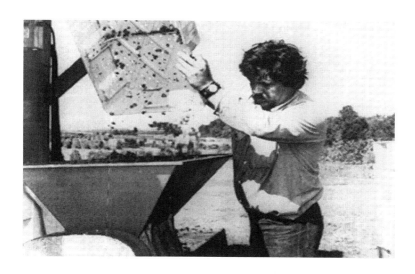

Len Olson was born on the south side of Chicago and eventually went to the University of Illinois on a football scholarship. Although he was injured and didn't play they won the Rose Bowl his senior year. His teammate was this guy named Butkus – hmmm, I think I've heard of him – yeah, Dick Butkus, NFL Hall of Fame...played for da Bears. "He went on to fame and fortune," Len said. "I went on to work in a non-profit career called making wine (laughing)."

He was a steel salesman whose territory included southwest Michigan. Also a self-taught winemaker, Olson actually did pretty good creating his own headlines in the Michigan wine industry in 1968. Among other eye-popping things, he planted the first commercial plot of European variety wine grapes in the state.

With his partner Carl Banholzer, they grew 27 varietals on Banholzer's 45-acre farm located on Mt. Tabor Rd. in Buchanan. "I was looking to get out of Chicago," Len remembered. "It was an angry town back then and I needed to breathe. When I planted those vines, they all thought I was nuts. They said it was a crazy man's dream." That vineyard and crazy dream would become the Tabor Hill Winery, which was licensed in 1970 and opened for business in 1972.

In those early years, they made wine the old fashion way – they stomped those grapes into juice. Business was rolling along but financial problems forced Olson to sell Tabor Hill in 1979. He left the winery and Michigan in 1982 to become a founding member of the Kentucky Wine and Grape Council.
He returned to Michigan 'because I had unfinished business' and started the Baroda Founders Wine Cellar in 2009. "I wanted to create a variety of wines for all palates," Olson recalled. "They range from the classic European varietals to one of his most popular red wines called *Oh Hell Yeah*.

As the story goes, Len came in from salmon fishing on the St. Joseph River and everyone was celebrating his catch with some rather expensive French Merlot. Len's friend Red set his glass aside saying 'don't like the stuff.' So Olson went to his car and fetched some juice just harvested from the Founders vineyard. After taking a sip, Red proclaimed 'oh hell yeah' and a new wine was born.

His wines have been served from the White House to Hollywood but he's just as happy serving visitors a glass of his latest creation from the Founders tasting room in Baroda, Michigan. There's a story behind every wine.

Interview with Len Olson:

Originally, when you were scouting land in southwest Michigan, was there really a Tabor Hill?

Len: The property is on the corner of Hill Road and Mt. Tabor. We thought the combination would work better than trying to use our names. When we tried to combine my partner's name, Banholzer, with Olson it came out sounding like a toilet bowl cleaner or deodorant.

Tell us about your first grape crushing experience.

Len: We made about 400 gallons in 1969, which was the homeowner's limit at the time. We tried to use a hand crank but it was taking a long time, so we just drilled holes in some half-barrels and started stomping with our feet. The wine turned out great. We maintain the tradition with our annual Grape Stomp on the Saturday after Labor Day.

In those early years, did you seek advice from other winemakers?

Len: I thought it was prudent to see how the best winemakers were doing things. I first went to California and talked with Robert Mondavi. He told me 'it's a shame you'll never be able to make good wine in southwest Michigan but we did look at that area to buy oak because it has some of the best American oak in the U.S.' I mentioned to him that the great oak forests of Europe were all located very near the great wine regions – why wouldn't it work in Michigan? His response was 'I can't tell you anything – go talk to my German winemaker consultant.'

And you did…with Kurt Werner and Helmut Becker, two renowned winemakers. What did you learn from them?

Len: Werner came to visit me and said 'Olson, you're like the one-eyed man in the land of the blind – you think you're King, but I will open both your eyes.' And he did by telling me the advantages of using a centrifuge to make wines clean and crisp. He introduced me to Helmut who was Head of the Geisenhiem Oenological and Viticultural Institute in Germany (grape and wine research). The most notable thing I learned was how they never use sugar to sweeten anything – they use grape juice with higher sugar content.

Do you remember the first bottle of wine you sold?

Len: (laughing) The absolute first bottle of wine I sold was on a Sunday, when Sunday sales were illegal, to my cousin who was a minor, after hours. But I think the statute of limitations is up – that was about 40 years ago. What I remember was working so hard to get the winery open and sitting around waiting and nobody showing up. So I started banging on doors and hitting the road to get the word out that we were open. I burned up the road between Detroit and Chicago making 12 to 15 calls a day back then.

Gerald Ford played an important role in getting the Tabor Hill name out there. Tell us about that.

Len: Peter Stroh of the Strohs Brewing Co. and Joe Muer of Muer's Restaurant fame in Detroit came to the winery with their wives. Peter's wife Nicole loved our Demi-Sec wine, which she said tasted like wine from her home in France and they took eight cases home. About two weeks later, I was sitting down to lunch and mentioned 'wouldn't it be cool if Pete and Joe got their buddy Gerald Ford to serve our wine in the White House? I no more said the word House and the phone rang. The guy said he was the Chief of Protocol from the White House and I thought it was one of my friends giving me a line of BS...but it really was him. President Ford was giving a speech the next day in Detroit so I loaded up 28 cases of wine, drove them to Metro Airport and I watched'em put it on Air Force One. I make basically the same wine today and it's called *Luce Del Sole*.

You had considerable success in the Kentucky wine industry. How would you compare Kentucky wines to Michigan wines?

Len: Kentucky wines are more like California wines. Our growing season is very much like Europe's. We can get 90-degree days but it goes back down to 70 at night. In Sonoma, they'll get over 100 during the day and only down to 90 at night. Kentucky doesn't get as hot but is similar with 95/80 temperatures. Our area enjoys the tempering effect from Lake Michigan, which makes our wines much easier to finesse. It makes for a gentler ripening and higher quality grape.

How did you come up with the Baroda Founders Cellar name?

Len: First, the Cellar is in Baroda and originally, I got the first winery license that wasn't grandfathered in after Prohibition. I've been recognized as the founding father of the premium wine industry in the Midwest.thus the name Founders. I take great pride in that but, in fact, that gets you one phone call, if you have fifty cents and can find a phone booth (laughing).

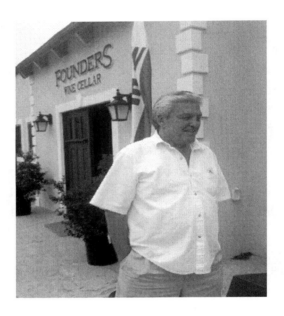

Your tasting room for the Founders Cellar is unique – what's the history of the building?

Len: It was a Buick Dealership back in the 50's and then a warehouse. Before we bought it, they used it to store boats and RV's. We cleaned it up and put a big long tasting bar in. There are lots of tables and historical pictures on the walls. There are windows behind the bar so you can view the wine production facility. It's a cool place to relax and enjoy some wine with friends.

I see your wine philosophy is 'drink in health.' What does that mean to you?

Len: I just think it's a nice saying – think about it – you can drink for your health or drink while you're healthy.

Here's to your health – long may the winemaker live – thanks Len.

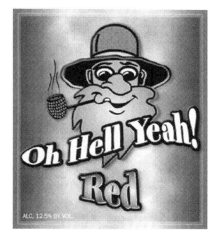

See Barodo Founders' ad on page 394.

CASCADE WINERY
The Urban Legend

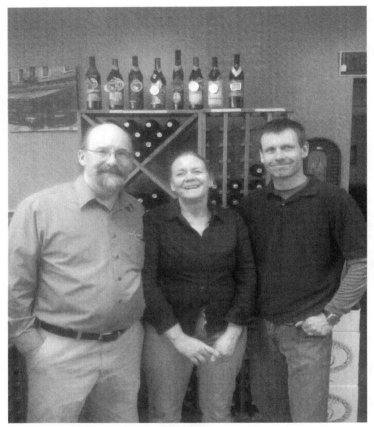

Cascade – Bob, Rose, and Roger Bonga

Bob and Rose Bonga don't mind working hard – it's just better when you're working for yourself. They were looking for something to do in their retirement years. So they took their hobby of making wine and created Cascade Winery right in the heart of the Grand Rapids' industrial south end. The hard work continues but the good wines they produce make it all worthwhile.

They took a 2,000 sq. ft. building at 28th St. and Cascade Rd. and converted it into an urban winery in 2003. The first thing they did was hire their son Roger. Originally, he was the all-everything guy while his parents continued working full-time at Amway Corp. Now Roger serves as the main winemaker and brew master for the JJ Brewery, which is also owned and operated by the Bonga family.

Bob continued with both jobs for two more years before retiring the 'working for the man' job. By then Cascade Winery was bursting at the seams and desperate for additional working space. "It's surprising how much more productive you can be when you don't spend a lot of time and energy moving things around," chuckled Bob.

In 2008, they moved into a 6,800 sq. ft. building on Broadmoor Ave. and added the brewery to the business. Once again, production exceeded available space so 4,000 more sq. ft. was utilized in 2012.

The winery portfolio also continued to grow with a selection of reds, whites, fruit and specialty wines. Regarding their urban setting, Bob says 'I like to say we bring the fruit to the city so you don't have to go to the fruit.'

Interview with Bob Bonga:

Cascade: A series of small waterfalls...well, it is Grand Rapids but are there any waterfalls around here?

Bob: I don't think so but we used to live on Cascade Rd. and our first winery was on the corner of 28th and Cascade. When we were trying to come up with a name, it was originally going to be our initials RJB – Rose, Roger and I all share those three letters. But there was a similar company name in the corporate register. We were both working the 2nd shift (3 to 11) so there were quite a few midnight discussions with a glass of wine and popcorn. One night there must have been an 'aha' moment – let's call it Cascade Winery – it stuck.

Was it difficult starting a winery and still working full-time, especially the 2nd shift?

Bob: Actually, it worked out really well – I loved the 2nd shift. I'm an early riser so when we were building at the first location, I could get a lot done in the morning when I was still fresh and had lots of energy. I'd go to work feeling good about what was accomplished and there was still time after my shift to kick back and relax at home before going to bed.

As an urban winery, the fermentation and bottling takes place here and you have the fruit shipped in…where does it come from?

Bob: From year to year, the wine we make is 80-90% from Michigan grown fruit/grapes. All of our fruit wines are from Michigan; all the whites except Muscato are Michigan grown grapes and four of our reds come from Michigan grapes – the rest are from California. We are having them shipped in and it's amazing how fast they get here. The grapes are picked in the morning, chilled and trucked to our facility in just over 48 hours – arriving in wonderful shape. It's nice to have some of those different varietals that you can't get here and it's always good to keep contacts out there in case we have bad weather here.

Many of your wines are closed with a screw cap. When did you start using them and were you pleased with the result?

Bob: We originally used cork for everything but went to screw caps for our fruit wines last year and will probably add the whites this year. We'll see in a few years about adding the reds. In my opinion, the screw cap as a stopper is superior to any other closure. Having said that, there is a shortage of screw top bottles because of the demand. The industry is starting to catch on.

One of the features at Cascade Winery is also having a brewery as well. Why and when did that happen?

Bob: A few friends in the industry had added a brewery to their facility and were very pleased with the results. It's a good fit and provides diversity, much as adding spirits to your portfolio, which we plan to do in the near future. When we moved to our new location, we just added more paperwork and applied for a brewing license as well. I tell people it's just as easy getting a license for a brewery, as it is a winery (laughing).

I'm not sure if that laugh was sarcastic or sadistic. So, outside of the paperwork, what was difficult about starting a winery and/or brewery?

Bob: We didn't start with a pot of gold so buying the equipment, which is quite expensive, was a challenge. Rose and I started all this with our 'nest egg' money so we've had to grow slow...neither one of us have a desire to go back to the real world and work full-time for 'the man' to keep this going.

You are basically a self-taught winemaker. Did Roger just learn from dad?

Bob: I did some reading, asked questions and experimented. Kids are more in tune with the Internet. Roger Googles everything and has a ton more information than I ever dreamed of learning. In the last five years, Michigan State University and the Michigan Grape and Wine Industry Council have also made a concerted effort to further everyone's education. The Council is always being pulled in different directions but they do a fantastic job of promoting the wine industry in Michigan. I always encourage new wineries to become a member as soon as possible. They are a big help.

Would you ultimately like to grow your own grapes?

Bob: We bought five acres not far from here and I'd like to someday have a plot of grapes to work with. I'm still a few years away from retirement but I've got to have a reason to get up everyday and do something. Roger is doing great as the wine and brew master and Rose retired a few years ago so she has the front and tasting room handled – I really don't have that much to do around here now...is Rose looking at me (laughing)?

Oh, I think they'll keep you around a while longer. Thanks Bob.

CODY KRESTA VINEYARD & WINERY
Dogs, Cats and Wine Rule

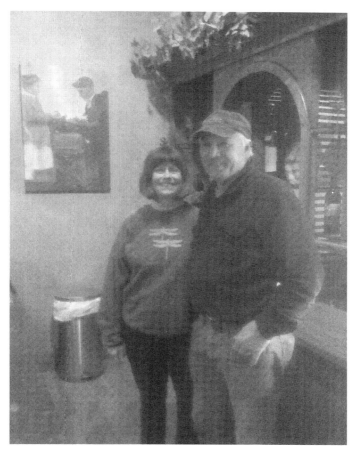

Wine dogs are commonplace in the wine world. But when you're greeted in the parking lot by a wine cat, who then leads you to the front door of the tasting room...that's a special place and David Butkovich makes special wine there as well.

Oh, there are dogs around and you quickly realize once the full story is revealed that dogs have played an important role in the Cody Kresta Vineyard and Winery ever existing.

You see, David's first golden retriever Sammy was a match maker – during a square dance in David's barn, the dog kept escaping the house and getting on Mary Lou's dance card – David finally got her telephone number, a marriage to the school speech therapist ensued and Sammy came with the deal. The winery is named after David and Mary Lou's second golden retriever, Cody (story to follow).

David's grandparents came from Croatia and settled in Mattawan to grow grapes for Welch's. Now, a third-generation winemaker, David has taken the skills he learned from working in his grandfather's vineyard and transferred them to his small family farm operation of 20 acres, with the goal of producing a low-volume of high quality wine grapes.

"We never really set out to build a winery," Mary Lou said. "We kept planting vines and making wine and eventually out produced our consumption. Every time a proverbial road block appeared an angel would magically make it disappear."

"Our intentions were to keep the operation small and have a quiet opening," David recalled. "A reporter came from the *Kalamazoo Gazette* to write about our new adventure. I thought it would make a nice 'filler' someday in the paper. It was on the front page the day we opened in June 2010. Remember in the movie Field of Dreams, 'build it and they will come' - we did and they did - in droves. We didn't even know how to run the cash register (laughing)."

A contractor by trade, David has built an efficient, beautiful facility out of the homestead 1882 barn with a patio out back overlooking the countryside – a perfect place to enjoy one of their twenty-three different wines and say hello to a few of the dogs and cats wandering about.

Interview with David and Mary Lou Butkovich:

How did you get the name Cody Kresta?

Mary Lou: Cody was our golden retriever dog and David's constant companion in the vineyard. One day a stray cat came by - Cody chased it out into the road and was killed. As a tribute, we thought of naming the vineyard after him.

David: Originally it was going to be Cody Ridge but with the Lawton Ridge Winery opening just down the road, we had to come up with something else.

Mary Lou: I thought it would be nice if we could somehow incorporate David's Croatian heritage into the name and a friend said 'hill in Croatian is kresta.' So our winery became Cody Kresta.

The logo is a beautiful likeness of your vineyard. How did that happen?

David: I came up with the script initials $\mathcal{C}$ $\mathcal{K}$ and we ended up superimposing the letters over the picture, which is the mural in our tasting room.

Mary Lou: We had a blank wall that originally was going to be covered with stonework. Then another one of those angels appeared. Our tasting room manager Leslie – who is our #1 Cody Kresta angel - suggested her neighbor, who is an artist, paint a mural and of course she painted Cody into the picture, as well.

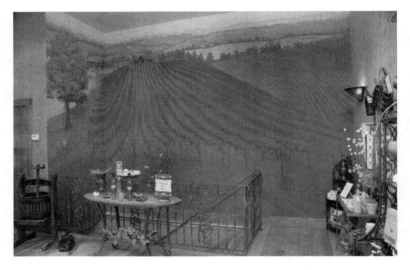

You've made multiple trips to California and Napa Valley. Did you try to pattern your wines in that style?

David: We both love Napa Valley dry wines and we thought that's what everyone would like.

Mary Lou: When we started telling other wineries what our plans were, everyone said you'll never survive on dry wines and they were right (laughing). David made a few sweet white wines but everyone was asking for a sweet red. Then David's father passed away a few years ago and his nickname was Rudy. So our first sweet red is called Rudy's Red and it flies off the shelf.

David: I can't tell you how many people tell me 'I don't like sweet red wines' and I'll just ask them to try a sip of Rudy's and they end up walking out with a case.

It is a small operation - how does the division of labor work?

Mary Lou: I handle everything on the computer and David handles everything else – brains and brawn (laughing). He's the oldest of seven siblings so he's got help available if needed. Every time we get ready to bottle, I start making the calls to friends and relatives. It would be difficult for David and me to do it all ourselves, so we've turned it into a big event. We buy pizzas and go into the house afterward – with plenty of wine, of course, and celebrate the new Cody Kresta vintage.

What is the most satisfying part for you as a winery owner?

David: The world in general can be very depressing at times and I think people just want to escape for a while. We work hard to create a friendly atmosphere and you can almost see the shoulders lift, the smiles come out – we've made a lot of new friends who like our wines, so we must be doing something right.

Do you draw a diverse crowd to your tasting room, i.e. tourists, travelers, in or out of state or mostly locals?

Mary Lou: It really is all of the above. So many of our customers comment about the serenity and quiet countryside out here but we're really only a few miles from I-94. Our road is paved but not real busy. We're not out in the boondocks…but we did get a couple who wanted a discount because we were 'so hard to find.' We'd never had anyone else complain about it before. So David gave them a discount.

David: Well, the customer's always right – even though they aren't sometimes, they're supposed to be (laughing).

For the most part, David, you're a self-taught winemaker but do you have a go-to guy?

David: I've worked with Chas Catherman, St. Julian's former winemaker, for four years now. He really knows his stuff. I remember our first year after we opened, we were taking a trip out to California and when we landed I received an urgent call from Leslie saying 'corks are flying everywhere' from our nice award-winning Rosé. While I started looking for a return flight to Michigan, I called Chas…he raced over to Cody Kresta to save the day. I was so embarrassed to tell anyone – then I found out later – it happens to every winemaker at one time or another (laughing).

As a farmer and contractor, you get to fix and build things. What's the history of your tasting room?

Mary Lou: It's unbelievable how many things can break at a winery. We built on because we needed the space and the tasting room was originally supposed to be my Tai Chi studio.

David: I should have doubled the space and if we continue to grow, I'll be doing just that.

Mary Lou: He kept nibbling until I just gave in and gave him the whole space but it's still the GIRL'S clubhouse after hours!

So, where do you see Cody Kresta in another five years?

David: We've nearly doubled in wine output each year – I'm very pleasantly surprised at how well we've done so far.

Mary Lou: We always said 'if it isn't fun anymore, we'll just lock the doors and drink up the inventory with our friends.' We keep making new friends who keep coming back to buy more wine and we're still having lots of fun.

Keep the doors open and we'll keep coming back – thanks to you both.

> See the Cody Kresta ad on page 401.

**This might be the wine talking,
but I think I want to order more wine.**

CONTESSA WINE CELLARS
Vino é Vita – Wine is Life

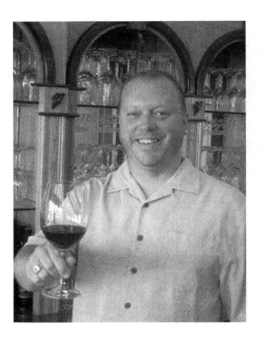

Tony Peterson grew up in Kalamazoo and began working in his father's vineyard by age twelve. It took many years before the wine grabbed his heart and got into his blood. Now looking out over his own vineyard and Contessa Wine Cellars, it is his life.

"The wine industry didn't seem as appealing at age twelve," chuckled Tony. "On a Saturday afternoon, I remember wishing I was playing baseball or football instead of picking fruit." After graduating from high school, Tony gave college a try but soon realized, working at the Peterson and Sons Winery wasn't so bad after all.

Although he gained valuable experience working for his father, by 2000 Tony was ready to take a leap of faith and venture out on his own. He purchased an old peach orchard in Coloma and began making plans for his own winery. "I started developing my own ideas about operating a tasting room and managing a vineyard," Tony said. "It was time to move on – so I went deep in debt and made it happen."

After building a chalet A-frame tasting room within eyesight of I-94, he opened Contessa Wine Cellars in 2002. "As much as I enjoy selling my wines, I enjoy selling the experience of tasting them as well. There are wonderful wines all over the world, including Michigan and right here in Coloma. It's more than remembering a good wine – I want visitors to remember the Contessa experience."

Sometimes it is the little things that make the experience memorable. On less crowded days, Tony brings out the crystal stemware, the bar stools feel comfortable, a fireplace makes the tasting room feel cozy on a winter day and the patio is a great place to view the vineyard on a summer day.

Even the wine list has added touches, like including the alcohol levels and residual sugar percentages – things that make the experience educational and enjoyable. "I describe it here as old world charm with modern amenities," he said.

Try his wines and get the 'Contessa experience' and you'll understand why Tony gets so many repeat customers.

Interview with Tony Peterson:

Where did the name Contessa and your wine label design come from?

Tony: Contessa is a family name and many of my wines carry that Italian theme – like my *Celeste* (heavenly), *Rosa d' amore* (rose of love) or the *Bianco Bello* (lovely white). I have a friend who is a graphic designer and I told her I wanted the image of a wine goddess looking into the vineyard holding a glass of wine – I think she nailed it.

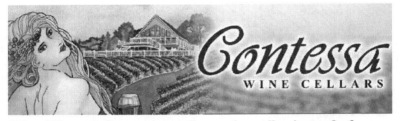

Why did you call your operation a wine cellar instead of a winery?

Tony: Originally, I thought it sounded more elegant. Hindsight is wonderful but immediately I ran into problems with people thinking I was offering a huge variety of wines like in a wine shop instead of just a selection from my vineyard. I would imagine it's the same problem with someone calling their place just a vineyard – in that case, people might not realize you also sell wine. Thankful, it's only been a minor problem.

Your slogan is 'Life is there – you just have to taste it.' What do you mean by that?

Tony: It is something I firmly believe in – you have to take whatever negative life deals you and spin it into a positive. Life is meant to be enjoyed – wine just makes it better.

What do you think makes Contessa wines unique?

Tony: I've taken a more traditional path by using more vinifera and making my wines drier. Most Michigan wine drinkers are used to a sweeter wine.

You have also put an emphasis on the 'wine experience.' What kind of experience can someone expect at Contessa?

Tony: We are striving to have visitors feel like they are walking into a home instead of a tasting room. Whenever possible, we use crystal glasses, which we hope makes it feel like a special occasion without being pretentious. Sometimes I think customers are expecting the hard sell to buy or get intimidated from lack of wine knowledge – we want them to feel just the opposite at Contessa.

Part of the elegance you have is using a special crystal stemware. Does it really make a difference?

Tony: It doesn't matter to some but it sets us apart, and to many it does make a difference. I use German Stolzle Crystal. It goes hand in hand with the presentation and perception of my wines. I do feel it enhances the flavors and aromas as well. Unfortunately, on those 'mad house weekends' we've had to resort to using more durable glassware to handle the crowds. We also serve Contessa wine by the glass out on the patio and crystal isn't practical out there on a windy day.

You also planted a Diamond grape in your vineyard. I'm not familiar with that varietal – where did it come from?

Tony: I think I'm the first to plant it in Michigan. I came across it in the Finger Lakes region of New York. The Diamond is a native American grape similar to the Niagara – white and typically makes a sweeter wine. We're looking forward to making wine with it – I think Contessa Diamond will be a big seller.

On your wine menu, you list residual sugar percentages. Most wineries don't – why is it important?

Tony: Each category of wine has a variation of sugar level. Of course, everyone's perception and taste is different. The residual sugar from 0-1 is a dry wine, 1-2 is semi-dry, 2-3 is semi-sweet and over 3 is a sweet wine. So, if someone says they prefer sweet wines there could be a big difference in the sugar levels of wines they actually like. It's another piece of information to help a wine drinker to hone in on what wines they enjoy and another way Contessa can educate our customers.

Many wineries offer chocolates or list wines that go well with chocolate. What's up with wine and chocolate?

Tony: First, who doesn't like chocolate (laughing)? Actually, I have met a few people in the last ten years who didn't care for chocolate but just a few! It's a wonderful pairing with many wines. I think they both have a tendency to heighten your taste buds. We have a sign next to our driveway – Wine here, Chocolate ½ mile. The Chocolate Garden is just down the road. Chocolate goes really well with our drier style wines.

Contessa Wine Cellars is on the Lake Michigan Shore Wine Trail and you're located right off I-94 – so you do have crazy wine weekends. How do you cope?

Tony: I love it when we're busy. There is almost a festive atmosphere in the tasting room. I'm always telling people to come back when it's less hectic because I love to spend time with them. Busy is nice but I also get a lot of satisfaction when there is just a couple in here with me learning about my wines. Wine is a wonderful subject to talk about.

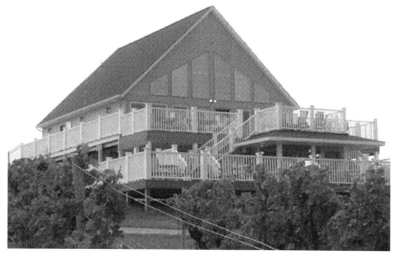

You are providing a wonderful source of enjoyment as well – thanks Tony.

See the Contessa Cellars ad on page 402.

DOMAINE BERRIEN CELLARS
A Little Rhone In Your Wine

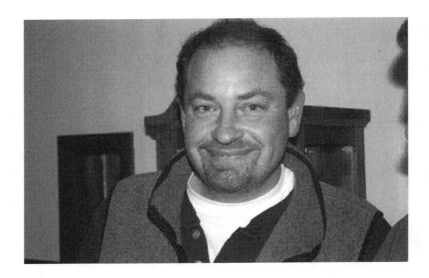

It was Wally Maurer's father-in-law, Tom Fricke, who envisioned the Rhone Valley of France in 1992 when he purchased an 80-acre cherry orchard in Berrien County. He had grown up in southwest Michigan and always wanted to grow grapes just like the French. Nine years later, that little chunk of Berrien County became Domaine Berrien Cellars.

Wally and Katie Maurer met in a Houlihan's Restaurant in Cleveland on St. Patrick's Day. "I was young and impressionable," chuckled Wally. "She was very impressive though because she converted an Irishman from beer to wine. After we married and were living in Chicago, we went to Michigan every weekend we could, escaping the city to help with the grapes and make wine at the in-laws."

Eventually, he took a severance package and began building the vineyard. "We began pulling out the old cherry trees and planting Rhone grape varietals," Wally said. "Tom was a visionary. He purchased one of the highest points in the county and knew with the right trellis system, you could have a well balanced vineyard, which in turn created great fruit and great wine."

When the vineyard was large enough to support a winery, they opened Domaine Berrien Cellars in 2001. Katie continued to commute until the winery was busy enough for her to make the move to Michigan permanently a few years later.

The vineyard now has twenty-one different varieties of grapes producing 100% estate wines. "Tom taught me to control your own fruit by making decisions in the vineyard, which will allow me to make the kind of wine I want to make before I ever taste it," Wally said.

Domaine Berrien Cellars offers eighteen different wines. "There's something for a Sommelier to try, something for the beginners and some I call 'transitional' wines for those wine lovers trying to educate their palates."

So let us take some time for Wally to educate us.

Interview with Wally Maurer:

How did you get the name Domaine Berrien Cellars?

Wally: First, we're in Berrien County. And the word *domaine*, in a loose interpretation, was the working man's farm in the

French countryside – unlike the chateaus of Bordeaux that had staff work the vineyards – we get our hands dirty.

Your label is unique and colorful. Who designed it?

Wally: Katie and I designed it – taking a bunch of ideas we both had – she's an engineer and I'm the artist, which you can imagine creates its own set of problems (laughing). I'm proud of the classic style with our name in script superimposed over the state of Michigan. We feel it's a reflection of our wines.

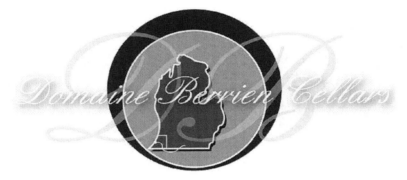

Your slogan is 'High quality grapes into high quality wine.' Is that more or less the heartbeat of your winery?

Wally: We like to start with quality and finish with fun. We're all about people enjoying our wines and enjoying the time here at the winery. We try to educate and entertain – it's all about the experience.

You grow a wide variety of grapes (21). What is the most difficult and why?

Wally: The Pinot Noir is difficult but my passion is growing the Cabernet Franc – it's a delicate but fickle grape. Midwesterners are starting to catch on to it and it's become quite popular.

Domaine Berrien is also environmentally certified by the Michigan Ag Environmental Awareness Program. Is that a fancy way of saying you're more "green"?

Wally: I'm all for being green if it will sell more wine (laughing). That's a little tongue in cheek – actually, it means we are demonstrating more stewardship in protecting the land, the ground water and surroundings through our planting, maintaining and harvesting practices. The word 'green' is the in-vogue word – those of us who've been around a while want sustainable agriculture, which means if you take care of the land, the land will take care of you.

Tell us about Steelhead White, Wolf's Prairie Red and your Crown of Cabernet.

Wally: The St. Joseph River runs through Berrien County and it has world-class steelhead trout in it. The wine is 'steely', clean and crisp (as I knock on my cool stainless steel tank). The Wolf's Prairie is named after a Potowatami Indian Chief Big Wolf – this was his territory. The Crown of Cabernet is my wine – blended just the way I like it. I'm just glad everyone else likes it to.

You host an Art, Wine & Music Festival (2013 is the 9th annual). How did it get started?

Wally: The festival has grown each year – we've maxed out on artist space, the music gets cranked up, we put the white on ice and the reds in the shade and have a great time.

What's the strangest question you've been asked at the winery?

Wally: There are a lot of big cities within easy driving distances – Detroit, Chicago, Fort Wayne…so we get a lot of 'city folks' coming to the country. One of them asked me if we had schools for our children to go to – I guess that person didn't get out much. Another time, we had a party and offered hay rides. A young lady said 'this is so much fun, do you do this every night?' We're just a couple kids from the sticks (laughing). We don't know nothing about business, just how to make wine and how to have fun.

You also have a couple wine dogs.

Wally: My black lab, Baco Noir, has been with me since we opened the winery. My mother-in-law said 'absolutely no puppies around here while you're trying to open a winery and living in my house' – Baco finally wore her down. We didn't know we needed a second dog but Mocha knew we did – he's a rescue dog that came home with Katie one day. He's a blend of about 50 different wine dogs. Baco likes the reds and Mocha likes the whites.

On your website, people have posted where they've taken a bottle or two of Domaine Berrien Cellars wine 'around the world.' Where are some of the more distant places?

Wally: We've had people send us pictures with our wine in New Zealand, Key West, Mexico, Hawaii – we even had a couple toasting our wine in the Coliseum in Rome. They must have smuggled it on to the airplane. I don't want people to get into trouble but I thought it was cool.

We'll send you a picture from Coleman, Michigan – that's a fairly remote place – thanks Wally.

The other day someone told me you could make ice cubes out of leftover wine. I was confused. What's leftover wine?

FENN VALLEY
A Legacy of Leadership

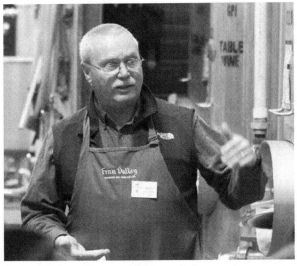

A lumberman and a science teacher – father and son – came to Michigan to set roots deep enough to become a cornerstone in the wine industry. From their farm in the little town of Fennville in southwest Michigan, Bill and Doug Welsch started the Fenn Valley Winery, which is now one of the largest wineries in the state and was built primarily by helping other wineries succeed.

"This all started as a hobby that got out of hand," Doug said. "Our family made wine and so did I, from the time I was a kid and I haven't stopped yet."

Bill Welsch had a successful lumber business on the south end of Chicago but by his late 40's he was growing bored and restless. "My dad was a Depression era survivor, who always thought the economy could crash again," Doug recalled. "He felt agriculture was the only secure form of investment. So that became his new challenge."

At that time, Doug was just finishing up college to become a science and biology teacher. The wine industry was just beginning to take off in the U.S., so he and his father began touring and talking to the early post-Prohibition pioneers of this new industry. They met with people from the Bully Hill Vineyards in the Finger Lakes region of New York, visited Napa Valley, which was just emerging, and went to visit the fledgling Tabor Hill Winery in Michigan.

While Doug was finishing school, Bill was searching for the right site to grow wine grapes. He settled on southwest Michigan and in 1973, he acquired two 80-acre farms adjacent to each other in Fennville. Doug moved on to the property in June of that year. "This is where it all started," Doug remembered. "They were old fruit farms. We cleared them off and started with bare ground."

His father acquired another 80-acres the next year, so with 240 total acres of prime fruit ground, they began planting hybrids and two vinifera – Riesling and Gewurztraminer. About half the vines didn't pan out. "I approached the business with a pragmatic attitude," Doug said. "I've always gone with what worked for us rather than the dogma that would dictate what we were supposed to do. It's always worth it to experiment and think outside the box a little."

Fenn Valley initially offered fruit wines. "If it grew in Michigan, I made wine from it," chuckled Doug. When the vineyards started maturing, they moved into grape wines. Today they still offer a few fruit wines but the majority are hybrids and vinifera. "My approach was not to make your second bottle until you sold your first."

They opened the Fenn Valley Winery in 1976 and the early years were rough. "We didn't get much respect here or anywhere," Doug said. "I'll tell you when it all turned around. In the early '90's, the show 60 Minutes had a segment called the "French Paradox"about the health benefits of drinking wine. All of a sudden wine was in – it was good for your health to drink wine."

They never looked back. Today, Fenn Valley is thriving with thousands of visitors every weekend touring the vineyards and tasting their award-winning wines.

Interview with Doug Welsch:

Your father learned from his father – what did you learn from your father?

Doug: I learned what not to do (laughing). To be honest, the wine was pretty awful at home. My dad was a home winemaker but really his forte was business. I was the scientist – we truly had an Ernest & Julio Gallo relationship. I was responsible for the winemaking and my dad was in charge of the business and marketing end. We had a great symbiotic relationship. He loved to push a pencil and I loved getting my hands dirty.

One of Fenn Valley's brochures says 'fine wines are made in the vineyard.' What is your take on that?

Doug: Most wineries take people through the production area. I had the entire farm licensed as a tasting room so we could sample wines out there. We take wagonloads of people out to where the wine is made. The winery is where you convert grape juice into wine. But the quality of that juice is made from the hard work in the vineyard. The ceiling for the quality of wine is already established before the winemaker goes to work.

You mentioned a willingness to experiment with different varieties. So is there a particular variety of grape or wine you are most proud of?

Doug: Yes, the newest and the one I'm most enamored with is Sauvignon Blanc. Whether or not it will be viable in the long run is yet to be determined because it's a difficult grape to grow. When the vine survives our winters, the wines are absolutely stunning. The old workhorse grape the industry has done well with is Riesling – that put us on the map.

Many wineries mentioned you for your willingness to help get them started. What advice do you give new winery owners?

Doug: I work with them in three primary areas. First, is picking the varieties that will grow in their ground and be commercially accepted by the consumer. Second, is equipment – I've made a lot of mistakes and wasted money on the wrong equipment, so I can help them avoid that. And third, is cash flow. A new winery has a lot of money tied up for years before they can get everything rolling. We can help with product until they can stand alone. In some cases, we've continued on with a working relationship and others have gone on to thrive without us. We want them all to succeed and sell good quality wine because everyone knows when you like something, you'll tell someone else, but if you have a bad experience you'll tell three people.

Name three turning points in Fenn Valley's history.

Doug: In 1991, I took over running Fenn Valley. That year we switched our marketing strategy from wholesale to retail. Then in the late 1990's, we started to schedule vineyard tours, which has had a huge impact and what we're known for today. It is an educational experience. And the third – I'll get back to you because I don't think it's happened yet but something will come up.

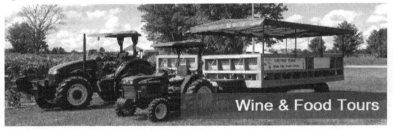

You were instrumental in getting the first American Viticulture Area (AVA) designation in Michigan. Why was that important?

Doug: During that time, if you vintage dated wine it had to have an AVA – a designated origin. The term 'American' wasn't allowed on labels back then and you couldn't use 'political' boundaries, i.e. Allegan County or Michigan. That's all changed now but then everyone was scrambling. Also, at the time, none of the Michigan wineries were talking to each other. They'd chat if they met on the street but in a meeting they couldn't agree on anything. So my father filled out the paperwork to apply for our own AVA. The Washington big wigs flew into west Michigan for a hearing and nobody showed up except me, my dad, a local historian and Chas Catherman from St. Julian to speak on our behalf. It was a big joke and was over in about 30 minutes. We were only the third AVA issued in the country.

As the 'wagon master' giving tours, what is the most surprising thing a visitor learns about Fenn Valley?

Doug: I think the most surprising thing they learn is how much work it takes to maintain a productive vineyard. When I tell them everything they see will be cut down in the fall, they're flabbergasted. They think we have an army of workers but they don't understand if you do the same thing everyday, it's the tortoise and hare scenario – we get it done because we keep at it.

What is Fenn Valley's wine philosophy?

Doug: We want wine to be available and affordable to the masses and not be an elite beverage. So I do everything possible to economize without sacrificing quality and pass that savings on to the consumer.

In your opinion, what makes a good vintner?

Doug: One word covers it all – passion. Most winemakers aren't professionally trained. They've learned how to make wine just like me, through trial and error. If there's no passion, you won't put up with the long hours. You won't put up with the variables you can't control – like having the best season ever, followed by the coldest season that you have to fight to survive. Passion is what gets you through.

What do want your legacy to be in the wine industry?

Doug: I just want to be known as a significant contributor to the birth of the industry – whether it is from the selection of grapes, making wines or helping to get other wineries started.

If there were a last supper for you, what would your food and wine pairing be?

Doug: It would be a nice dark chocolate with a big glass of Cabernet Franc.

May that be many years from now and may I say I think your legacy is secure – thanks Doug.

See the Fenn Valley ad on page 403.

I've yet to meet a problem wine can't fix.

GLASS CREEK WINERY
Up The Creek With a Glass Of Wine

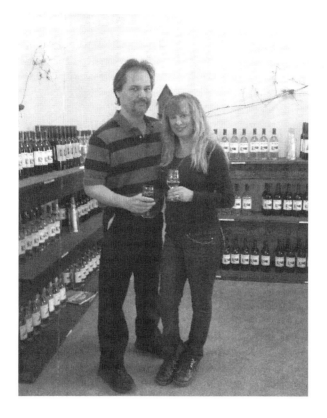

Eric and Donna Miller went from home winemaking to opening a winery, which isn't an easy process. They went from making wine in five gallon buckets to fifty-five gallon tanks, which is harder than you think. For a fledgling winery, getting a reliable fruit source is an uphill struggle.

Even after all these challenges, the Miller's opened Glass Creek Winery in August 2012 and they were very optimistic. They are certainly 'glass half-full' people and rightfully so because their customers keep coming back for refills.

They met while working for a Grand Rapids manufacturing company and the plan was to build their own winery just down the hill from their home near Hastings, Michigan. Donna took early retirement, 'I know I don't look old enough to retire (laughing)' and then served as the general contractor to oversee the construction of Glass Creek Winery.

Being the first and only winery in Barry County created a new set of problems to overcome but it has never been a problem making good tasting wine. Eric, who is the winemaker of the operation, has created a well-rounded wine list. He uses locally grown fruit sources, some out-of-state grapes and is adding Michigan suppliers where possible.

With construction complete and only six months of customer feedback, it's apparent their optimism has been rewarded judging by the number of wine glasses filled and the number of customers smiling as they take bottles of wine out the door.

Interview with Donna Miller:

So, there really is a Glass Creek?

Donna: You can see the creek from our tasting room patio. It actually flows right past our property, starting up at Thornapple Lake and eventually running back into the Thornapple River near Middleville. Eric and I came up with several possible names – one was White Pine because we have nearly 500 pines on our eight acres. We both like the Glass Creek connection because of its proximity, the natural surroundings and being a water resource of Barry County. Our labels, which have an artist's rendition of the creek, came from actual photos we gave to her to work from.

As one of the 'new kids on the block' in the Michigan wine industry, has it been difficult to procure a source for grapes?

Donna: Many of the growers already have contracts with other wineries and the grape supply is finite but we're using one Michigan grape already and are working with a few other Michigan growers to develop a reliable source of quality grapes. At this time, we are also bringing in grapes from Canada and Napa Valley.

What are you doing to get the word out about Glass Creek Winery opening its doors?

Donna: We're on the Pure Michigan website and will be added to the West Michigan Wine and Beer Trail this year. There are also quite a few festivals and events at the Barry County Fairgrounds, which is just down the road, so we're getting a lot of visitors from outside the area.

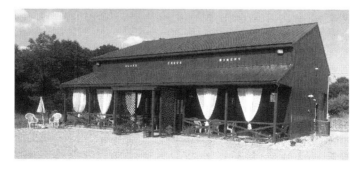

I understand the paper work can be a bit daunting in starting a new winery. What other hurdles did you have?

Donna: Three things immediately come to mind. First, I wanted to save some money so I was the general contractor for the building project. I will NEVER do that again for any project! Second, because there is alcohol involved, the FBI does a background check, so it was a little unnerving to have an FBI agent show up at the door – not that we had anything to worry about (laughing). And last, because we are the first winery in Barry County, many of the agencies were learning the red tape along with us and many times we would get contradictory information on what needed to be done. It was challenging just finding the right answers. Bob Bonga at Cascade Winery in Grand Rapids mentored us and was extremely helpful.

How did Eric decide which wines to make at first?

Donna: Originally, it was what you know, what you like and what you think will sell. Over time the wine list will solidify somewhat but right now it evolves. The wines that move we keep making and the ones that don't, get eliminated. What we've found is when one wine gets real popular, it naturally hurts the sales of other wines, so the goal is to offer a variety of grape and fruit wines that are fairly even in sales and popularity.

A wine drinker's palate usually evolves – did you ever think you'd be evaluating wine, trying to think what other people would like?

Donna: I never dreamed of owning a winery and never even drank wine until I was over fifty. In my 20's and 30's, I was strictly a beer drinker. Then in my 40's I switched to mostly mixed drinks. Now, its only wine and I leave the wine-making decisions up to Eric. He loves the whole process and I'm the designated wine taster.

Are there plans to eventually grow your own grapes and fruit?

Donna: Yes, we have already planted some Pinot Noir and Riesling varieties and several different fruit trees. All of our wines are made right here, which surprises a lot of customers. We're always being asked where the grapes come from and it will be nice to say they come from right here on our property.

What are your future plans to make Glass Creek Winery unique from others?

Donna: The plan is to have Eric retire in five years and expand to offer a larger variety of wines, maybe some sparkling wine and non-alcohol wines, and start up a microbrewery. One of the things that already make us unique is the country setting. People will come here just to sit on the patio, enjoy a glass of wine and watch the birds and wildlife. The deer are so used to them, they'll come right out of the woods to graze.

By the woods, by the creek, by the glass…thanks to the optimists at Glass Creek Winery.

GRAVITY WINERY
The Fun Will Pull You In

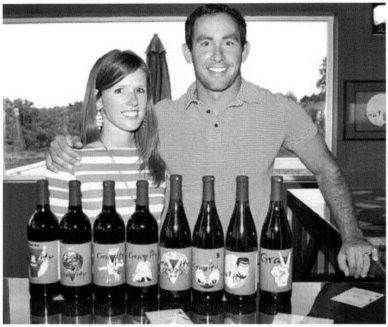

Just a few miles east of Baroda in southwest Michigan, in the heart of the Lake Michigan Shore Wine Country, you'll start feeling a force begin to pull on you. As it draws you closer, you'll see signs directing you to Gravity Winery.

When you start hearing the sounds of people having a good time, you begin to understand the effects of Gravity. That's exactly the effect owners Rockie and Allison Rick are trying to achieve at their winery.

Rockie grew up just down the road on a family farm that grew apples and peaches. After getting college degrees in agriculture and business, he began planting wine grapes in 1997, with the idea of eventually opening his own winery. "He was born to be a farmer but loves the office work as well," Allison said. "Being a vineyard and winery owner is the perfect business for him because I don't think he'd be happy at just one or the other."

He currently manages 40 acres of vines with 11 different grape varieties. Along the way he met Allison while they were serving as leaders for Young Life, a non-profit Christian youth organization. After they married, they started Fruitful Wine Tours and began saving up to build Gravity Winery. "The tour business was excellent research to find what the public liked and disliked about wineries," recalled Allison.

Gravity became a reality in 2011 as they began selling bottles of wine from small batches made on the premises of their current tasting room. It features a large patio overlooking nearly four acres of vineyard onsite, live music on Friday nights and wood fired pizza, paninis and appetizers from the Gravity Grill on weekends.

They serve 'flights' of wine with food pairings or wine by the glass from a list of thirteen different wines. But it's the labels that will catch your eyes first – each one is fun, unique and…catchy.

Interview with Allison Rick:

One of your goals is to 'put the fun back in wine.' How are you accomplishing that?

Allison: We think people used to go to wineries primarily to buy their supply of wine, whereas today they're visiting wineries for the experience and may or may not buy some wine. We're trying to cater to that philosophy and concentrate on the experience and making the wine sales secondary. At Gravity, we don't call it wine tastings – our samples are all with food pairings. We have a large sitting area inside and outside so we're not concerned about a fast turnover. The visitors can take their time. Even if they don't buy wine, we're glad they've had the chance to experience our customer service. It's a fun place to be.

So you are also the designer of Gravity's 'unusual' fun labels?

Allison: I make a sketch and send it to our legal guy who puts it on a computer.

But do you come up with the sketch before the wine is made or make the wine and come up with a sketch that fits it?

Allison: For most of our wines, you need a label approved by the time you are bottling it. So I have a stockpile of label concepts that we pick from to go with the wine before it's made.

Give us some examples of your 'whimsical' sketches that have become wine labels – all of them featuring a V.

Allison: Each label has a story – which, again, is part of putting the fun back in wine. Our Shiraz has a 'Bruce Lee looking' karate kid because the wine has a little kick to it. The Vacation Vino Blend is in a clear/frosted bottle to see the color of the wine and the label has two palm trees that form a V with the sunset in the background. Spock was actually my first label and no, I'm not a Trekkie. I just knew the guy made this hand sign that formed a V and it meant 'Live long and prosper.' That's exactly what we want for all the people who drink our wine.

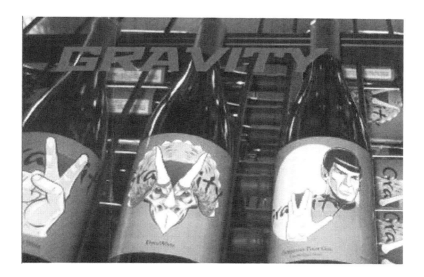

Your wine dog Oliver also has his own label but why does he have restricted access to the tasting room?

Allison: He's a great greeter but really he's an outdoor free-range dog. His label for Ollie's White is a picture of him wagging his tail while chasing a bird – one of his favorite pastimes. People are always letting him in and then he's trying to get back out so we finally just posted an Oliver restricted access sign (laughing).

Can you share with us some of your future wine label concepts?

Allison: Actually, we are offering the opportunity for our customers to submit suggestions for our labels. We have plans to change two labels each year and this will be a chance for someone to have their idea seen on a bottle of Gravity wine.

Where did the name Gravity come from?

Allison: That's the original way wine was processed by way of a gravity flow system – basically, the raw product started at the top and juice ready to bottle came out at the bottom. We also hope that Gravity affects you in a positive way and continues to pull you back to the winery.

You serve your wines in 'flights.' What does that mean?

Allison: We serve four wines of your choice – red or white – about 1/3 of a glass for each wine. Reds are paired with chocolates and the whites are served with different cheeses. They each have a specific purpose to pull out and emphasize the characteristics of our wines.

Rockie once said he 'yearned to be his own boss.' What do you see as the advantage or disadvantage of that while owning a winery?

Allison: The advantage is being able to fix a problem as soon as it occurs. The disadvantage is the winery being on your mind 24/7. If we go out to dinner, we have a difficult time not talking about the winery. We're never off the clock but we also know our energies are going toward something we're very proud of.

Tell us about the Gravity Growers Vine Club.

Allison: You actually own one of the Gravity vines – a Cabernet Franc or Riesling, with your name on a plaque. Then we have four 'hands on experience' events throughout the year to check on your vine's progress. We use these times to educate our friends about vineyard management, plus they get a 30% discount on all purchases.

What's next for Gravity?

Allison: We'll be building a much larger production facility soon and then we're putting Rockie's great experience with apples to good use by planting some trees that are specifically cider oriented. So we'll be adding hard ciders to our offerings in the future.

Well, it's obvious to me that you are specifically oriented to making sure everyone has a good time at Gravity – thanks Allison.

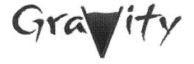

HICKORY CREEK WINERY
Old Ways – New Owners

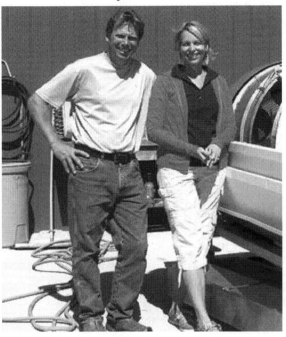

The Hickory Creek Winery of Buchanan was bought by Eric and Jayne Wagner in May 2012 – a fresh start for the winery that opened in 2006. The one holdover from the previous ownership is the winemaker, Mike de Schaff. The reason he's still there…the Wagner's love his wine and he does it the old fashioned way.

"Mike has a great reputation and we also wanted a smooth transition," Eric said. "Jayne likes Chardonnay and I'm a bold red wine drinker. The drier style winemaking already existed at Hickory Creek and we're staying committed to following that trend."

Jayne was born in Michigan but both she and Eric have called Chicago their home for many years. He's a veterinarian and she's in advertising. They also vacationed in southwest Michigan for many years and finally bought a second home nine years ago – a 33-acre property called Snow Hill Farm not far from the winery.

Eric sold his practice three years ago but still works there three days a week. When they heard about Hickory Creek Winery being for sale in 2011, the Wagners saw a new business opportunity.

Eric has an undergraduate degree in microbiology and had some experience with making beer and wine at home but nothing on the commercial level. The whole purchasing process took six months. "I've always known the wine industry is highly regulated," he said. "But when the FBI shows up to interview you and the local sheriff comes by to fingerprint you…it's kind of an eye-opener. I guess it all started from the Prohibition days."

No criminal element here – just bringing in a little of the Chicago way…wine drinking way that is. "We always liked Hickory Creek Winery's drier wines because it reminded us of what we and so many of our friends back in Chicago like to drink," Eric said.

They currently have a wine list with seventeen different offerings – something for everyone, including Rieslings, Apple Wine and Gewurztraminer.

Interview with Eric Wagner:

How familiar were you with Hickory Creek Winery prior to buying it?

Eric: We had been coming to taste and buy their wines for years. We also liked the name. People in the area identify with it, so we had no desire to change the name after taking ownership.

The label is very simple but has a unique design. What's the history behind it?

Eric: Again, it's something we liked about the winery. If you look close, the silhouette of the bottle is actually a three, which represents the three original owners. It was an American, an Australian and a German who started the winery back in 2006. Two returned to their home country and the American, Mike De Shaaf, stayed – he's the winemaker and was another reason we bought the winery.

What is your source of grapes for the wines?

Eric: We get all of our grapes from the Lake Michigan Shore AVA but Mike also has a good source from his own farm. Plus several neighboring vineyards are supplying grapes. Everyone is within a 10-mile radius of the winery.

On your website, you use the term 'vertical tasting.' What does that mean?

Eric: We make a Chardonnay wine and have different vintages. People may like one year better than another. Vertical tasting is lining up different vintages to do a comparison with each year.

There are subtle differences with the climate and quality of grapes that should come out with each vintage.

You also mention using 'old-world techniques' to craft wine. Could you explain?

Eric: We use European vinifera varietals and not hybrids or 'American' grapes. They all have French or German origins. The processes we use are basic – no refrigerated tanks, nothing is automated, we do cold soaks and techniques the French winemakers were using hundreds of years ago to get the taste we're looking for. It's not unique but we prefer a more hands on approach.

There is also a phrase on your website – 'Wine is bottled poetry.' That sounds like it came from someone in advertising rather than a vet.

Eric: That would be the work of Jayne and Mike. I'm the weed whacker guy (laughing). Jayne handles the social media, the marketing and helps Mike come up with those nice adjectives to describe wine. But each person's tastes are different as is each person's interpretation of poetry. Mike is the veteran on the team so we take direction from him and we work well together.

Prior to purchasing Hickory Creek Winery, did you have grapes growing on Snow Hill Farm and do you plan to have estate grapes there?

Eric: There actually are juice grapes growing there now and we're planting a plot of wine grapes in 2013 and will continue to expand the vineyards. It's expensive with the labor, the cost of the vines, the posts and wire but ultimately we want to use as much of our own grapes as possible.

You've already had a significant PR event with your wine being featured at a NATO summit meeting in Chicago – that was a nice perk.

Eric: Yes, that makes a nice talking point. We have several connections in Chicago and feel that area has great potential for our wines. It's been our experience that the wine drinking population in Chicago prefers a drier wine. Our tasting room sees many people from the greater Chicago area vacationing in southwest Michigan.

What aspect of owning a winery has appealed to you?
Eric: I come from a science background and although we've only owned the operation a short time, I've really enjoyed learning about the winemaking process – from the growing of the grapes to the chemistry to the bottling. I'll leave the selling aspect of the business to the others. My personality fits projects with a defined start to finishing point. The marketing and sales are more open-ended. That's Jayne's forte and she loves it.

People can also look forward to a new 'old' wine at Hickory Creek. Tell us about the Gruner Veltliner.

Eric: It's an old European grape (Austrian) that makes a wonderful white wine. Mike grows it on his farm and we think Michigan wine drinkers will love it.

No wine before it's time – we're looking forward to it – thanks Eric.

HOMETOWN CELLARS
Like Going Home

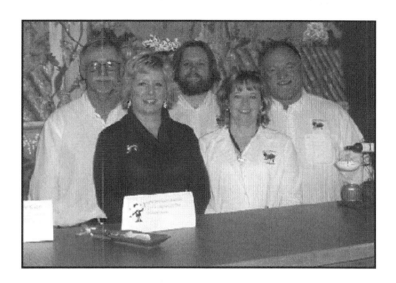

Take two brothers, two wives, throw in a son or two and you've got a hometown crew to operate Hometown Cellars Winery. Tom and Mindy Hale, with Ken and Terry Hale created a place to go for fun, relaxation and good wine or beer, just off US 27 right in downtown Ithaca.

"The family sweat equity is evenly distributed," said Terry. "Ken is a construction worker and Mr. Fix It. Tom is a car salesman so he handles outside sales, Mindy was a banker so her job is finance and the books and I am the people-person and worker bee (laughing)." Tom and Mindy's son, Aaron, is the winemaker and his brother is the brewmaster - truly an 'all in the family' operation.

Originally, the facility was meant to be a 'make your own wine' place and Hometown Cellars wine outlet. Opening in 2005, the Hales soon discovered their customers wanted to kick back and relax at the winery. So within a year, they expanded and began offering wine by the glass and appetizers. In 2008 they added the microbrewery.

The winery offers a selection of over 30 different wines ranging from $8-$20 and eight different craft beers. They also still offer the opportunity to make your own wine.

Interview with Terry Hale:

How did the Hales come up with Hometown Cellars?

Terry: We all sat around coming up with a list of names - it turns out wine and beer are good for the creative juices (laughing). Actually, Ithaca is our hometown and Tom, Ken and Mindy were all born and raised here, so with a downtown site the Hometown Cellars name made sense.

You were obviously using creative juices to come up with a label as well - tell us about that.

Terry: We originally just picked a label from a book and put our name on it. Eventually we wanted a more personal, professional looking one. A local artist came in and painted a mural in our winery and we all liked the idea of using it as a background for our new label. The sizing to make everything fit proportionally and making sure everything is proper and legal takes time - of course it all has to be approved as well. You wouldn't think it was all that difficult but a lot of time and energy was put into that label.

What was the most frustrating part of starting a winery?

Terry: For me, it was the waiting. You get everything in order, which entails a lot of work and then you wait for all of the paperwork to be approved and everything has to pass inspection. Then it's ongoing every time you change a label and when we added beer you start again - just like in the army - hurry up and wait.

All of the major players are family members - has that caused any problems?

Terry: If my sister-in-law has a voodoo doll of me at home, I haven't felt any needles poking my neck yet (laughing). Seriously, the family dynamics are always going up and down but we love each other and we're still here after seven years. The problem is everyone has an opinion but what makes it work is everyone wants the same thing, for this winery to succeed.

For you, what is the most satisfying part of this whole winery/microbrewery business?

Terry: Well, I am a purebred Irish woman, so I love sitting after work with a big cold pint of lager brewed by my nephew (laughing). But looking at the big picture, it is hearing the towns people say 'hey, we're coming to the winery tonight' or seeing my husband and brother-in-law having a great time serving customers from behind the bar or when people come in and want to meet the winemaker. We all take a lot of pride in producing wine and beer that people enjoy in a nice friendly and comforting environment.

Aaron the winemaker

He started with his first batch in 1998 from locally grown Concord grapes and like most beginners 'it was horrible.' He said, "winemaking and brewing began as an outlet from a natural curiosity about science and nature since he was very young.

"I actually have gotten to put some of my chemistry education to good use," Aaron chuckled. Eventually he gravitated from wine to concentrating on mead, while his father and uncle were producing grape wines and his brother experimented with home brewing beers.

As the winery started to shape up and Aaron was job prospecting, the family call came to entice him to return home.

How did the old winemaker take to the young guy coming in?

Aaron: Actually, it went very well - especially when I started proving my worth with contributions in laboratory skills like establishing environmental control and reproducing quality wines.

Do you have a 'go to' person when problems arise?

Aaron: I participate in a moderated Facebook discussion that's been going on for four years. It includes an excellent cross-section of professional winemakers and amateurs and is a collaborative effort with a great exchange of helpful information.

Is there a big difference in the fermentation process between

fruit wines and mead?

Aaron: Yes, the primary difference is yeast, which is used to convert sugar into alcohol, requiring some vitamins and minerals that are naturally present in fruit and grapes - they aren't present in honey, which is what mead comes from. So we give our mead vitamins to help the yeast get the job done. The other big difference is introducing oxygen prior to fermentation with mead and that's a no-no with wine.

Where do you see Hometown Cellars in the future?

Aaron: We've really remained stable during the economic downturn and have seen measurable growth in the retail markets. I think we'll continue to grow as the economy makes a comeback. It's interesting to hear people talk about their personal impact when the economy is down. They might reconsider buying a new car or remodeled the house or shift their investments but after talking about it for a while, it's 'man I need a glass of wine' (laughing).

I'll drink to that - thanks Aaron.

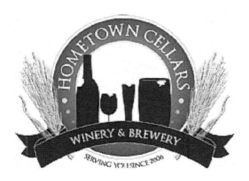

KARMA VISTA WINERY
Destiny With A View

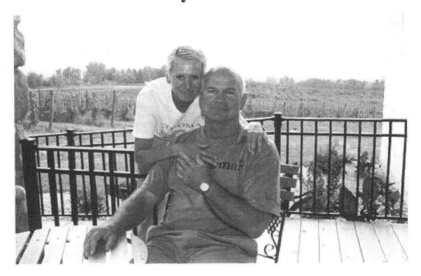

The path to Karma Vista Winery for Joe Herman started back in 1847 when his family settled in Coloma to grow fruit. Joe is the sixth generation to carry on the business but the first to add wine grapes and start a winery. It was meant to be.

One of six children, Joe was told by his father to get an education and get off the farm. "I did what my father wanted – I went away to college and got a four-year degree in journalism at Marquette University in Milwaukee," he said. "My first job was ten miles down the road as a reporter for the Benton Harbor newspaper – first assignment – the farm page."

It took only a year before he returned to the farm. By 1986 Joe was in charge of the 275-acres of fruit and then 'everything went to hell.' The only bright light, as the wholesale fruit market crashed, the major juice company Welch's was expanding. So Joe started growing juice grapes to supplement the peach and cherry orchards. By 1999, they added wine grapes to sell to other wineries.

The Herman orchards are also a prime retail location only a few miles from 1-94. Creating a winery was a natural step forward. "I looked at other wineries in Indiana, Ohio and New York," Joe said. "None of those areas are as gifted with climate conditions as we are right here in southwest Michigan. So I started planting vines at the bottom of the hill and figured when I got to the top, I'd build a tasting room."

He did reach the top and opened Karma Vista Winery in 2002. Several factors made the winery a success from the beginning. They grow quality grapes, which has turned into quality wine and the campaign to 'eat and drink' locally really helped. "We also have a large population to draw from," Joe said. "A 3-hour driving radius includes Detroit, Indianapolis and Chicago – something like 17 million people. If we just serviced the wine drinkers in that population, we couldn't grow enough grapes."

Karma Vista celebrated their 10th anniversary in 2012 and by the size of the crowds gathering in their tasting room, they may have to plant more grapevines.

If you are looking for a Zen moment with a nice wine and amazing view – Karma Vista is the place.

Interview with Joe Herman:

Did you have an 'Aha! moment' in deciding to start a winery?

Joe: It actually was more like a Homer Simpson D'OH! moment. In 2000, there was a meeting at one of the southwest Michigan wineries (there were only three at the time – Lemon Creek, Round Barn and Tabor Hill – now there are over thirty) and they emphasized only getting into the wine business if you can sell directly to the customer, which requires a good retail location. I was thinking about buying a site as I was driving home. About that time, I came around the bend heading east on I-94 and I'm staring at my 90-acre hill. My next thought was 'Joe, you idiot, you've already got the site.'

Was the transition from juice grapes to including wine grapes that difficult?

Joe: That's interesting because I would go to juice grape growers meetings and they would all say 'you don't want to grow wine grapes because you need a good retail site' and I'd say I've got one…then it was 'you don't want to do that because it takes a lot of people' and I'd say I've already got the people. Then they bring something else up and I'd say 'is it worse than growing peaches?' – 'Oh, no, it's not worse than peaches.' Well, I was already growing peaches. It couldn't be any worse.

So what inspired Karma Vista?

Joe: My wife Sue and I always loved the view up there, so the name was going to be 'something' Vista. I've got a minor in philosophy and at the time I was very fatalistic about this new venture – this was our karma or it wasn't. The western culture has always taken the eastern culture and bastardized it and I've always said karma was the great things that happen from the little things you do. We learned at a conference that most people couldn't remember the name of a winery one week after visiting it, so I've always claimed our name is part metaphysical, part Madison Avenue. The only problem with our name is people come in asking if we're Buddhist.

You have also used a little flair in writing the name.

Joe: We had this idea of extending the K to go out and comeback to dot the i, the way karma comes back to you like a wonderful little gift. For some reason, the artist kept wanting to make it look like a shooting star. Finally I just put a piece of tracing paper over his drawing and did it myself – then he had his A'ha! moment. That's the script version…the latest is putting a dove on the end of a wine bottle – a blatant Woodstock rip-off we added to our Peace, Love & Wine series.

So you're bringing back your hippie mojo?

Joe: Yeah, baby. Woodstock was about 'the times, they are a changin.' There is so much turmoil out there and people just want to get away from it for a while. That's what our Peace, Love & Wine theme is all about. We want to send out a good vibration to attract people.

You do use a lot of rock n roll references and lyrical quotes. Do you have a favorite?

Joe: My favorite is Bob Dylan's All Along The Watchtower – 'businessmen, they drink my wine, plowmen dig my earth, none of them along the line know what any of it's worth.' So many wineries are started by millionaires who know nothing about growing grapes and we are grape growers who know nothing about being millionaires. The bottom line isn't important to some wineries and at many wineries a $2 difference in price keeps them in business. Most people don't realize how much labor, time and money goes into each bottle of wine.

There seems to be an endless supply of clever names on your wine bottles. Who is the creator?

Joe: Blame only me...usually late at night, a wine induced name comes to me. There are still a few names I have to create a wine for. We just recently bottled some wine from our Marquette grapes, so I've given a nod to my University – if nothing, I should be able to sell it to the alumni.

What's the funniest thing you've been asked in the tasting room?

Joe: Well, the tasting room is way up on the hill and from Ryno Road visitors take a long winding drive through rows of grapevines on both sides up to the parking lot. Once there, you have a beautiful panoramic view of the vineyards. They come inside and ask 'where do you get your grapes?'

Is there any final piece of advice from the philosophical winemaking rocker from Coloma?

Joe: To quote the rock group Yes – 'don't surround yourself with yourself.' We baby boomers probably quote rock lyrics more than Shakespeare or the Bible. If Bob Dylan were alive during that time he may have become one of the missing books.

In the words of Bob Dylan, 'may your heart always be joyful and may your song always be sung – may you stay forever young.' Thanks Joe.

Karma Vista VINEYARDS

See the Karma Vista ad on page 409.

LAWTON RIDGE WINERY
A Nice Pairing of Partners

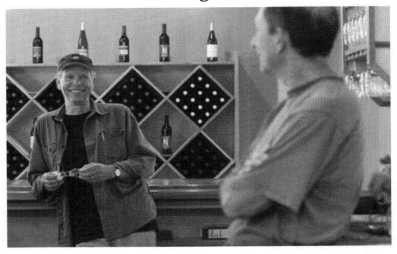

Dean Bender is a chiropractor and Crick Haltom was a chef. They formed a partnership through a love of wine and it became Lawton Ridge Winery, just fifteen minutes from downtown Kalamazoo.

"I was in Dean's office one day back in 1995," Crick recalled. "We had discussed wine many times but on that particular day he said 'I'm bottling wine this weekend – would you be willing to help?' and we haven't stopped since."

Dean, a native of Marshall, was an owner in the Lawton Ridge Vineyard and had become their winemaker (headquartered in his garage). Crick, a southerner from Mississippi, moved to Kalamazoo (because he and his wife loved the area) and has been involved in the food industry most of his adult life as a chef, a baker and vegetable farmer.

It became more than just making wine as a hobby – they shared a passion to make fine wines. Their first commercial wines, with the assistance of the Fenn Valley Winery, came in 2007. "The staff at Fenn Valley was very helpful and Doug Welsch has been a great mentor to us," Crick said.

After an initial thought of building a tasting room on the vineyard site, they bought a building on Stadium Hwy. between Kalamazoo and Paw Paw, opening for business on Aug. 1, 2008.

Lawton Ridge is the most eastern winery on the Lake Michigan Shore Wine Trail and many of their customers are heading west on I-94 from southeast Michigan and northern Ohio. Because you can't see any vines from their parking lot, Crick is asked all the time 'where do your grapes come from and where's the vineyard?' "Even the out-of-staters are pleased to know much of our fruit source is homegrown," Haltom said.

They currently offer fifteen wines including their 2010 Best of Class, AZO semi-dry red and their 2011 Late Harvest Vignoles, which won the 2012 Tasters Guild Trophy for Best Dessert Wine.

Obviously, the partnership is working.

Interview with Crick Haltom:

I have to ask – is there really a Lawton Ridge?

Crick: I'm not sure if it has an official name but yes, there is a hillside near Lawton that has the name Lawton Ridge Vineyard. The vineyard was started by several professors from Western

Michigan University back in 1970's – its actually south and west of here about seven miles south of the Paw Paw exit off I-94. The locals get confused because there actually is a town of Lawton. Juice grapes have been grown in that area for over 100 years.

What inspired them to grow grapes for wine there?

Crick: I believe one of the professors was making trips to France and sending back bottles of French wine to his friends and the light bulb came one - they thought 'we should be doing this ourselves.' So they bought an old peach orchard and planted two acres with twenty different varietals. There are about 10 acres planted now.

How much of your grapes come from the Lawton Ridge Vineyard?

Crick: About 80% of our wine is made from grapes grown there but we determined some red varietals, like Merlot and Cabernet Sauvignon, probably wouldn't do well there because it's a bit too far from the lake. The other 20% of our fruit still comes from southwest Michigan.

You have some beautiful paintings on your wine labels – who is the aviation nut and what does AZO mean?

Crick: Neither one of us is into aviation. AZO is the call sign for the Kalamazoo airport and we do have a friend, Rick Herter, who is an aviation artist. He was interested in doing some art for our labels. We came up with the name AZO Red for a new semi-dry red wine we had, which was so successful we later added an

AZO White – that required another one of Rick's paintings. Ironically, the yellow plane is on the red wine label and the red plane is on the white wine label.

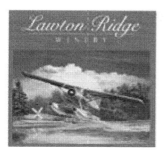
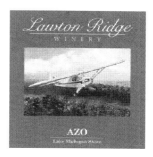

In your partnership with Dean, what assets does each of you bring to the winery?

Crick: Dean is a superb winemaker and runs the back end…I run the front as the business manager. Dean is a harsh critic when evaluating his own wines and I'm closer to the consumer's taste. So I'm the one usually saying 'it could be different but would it be better?'

Tell us the history of your building.

Crick: It's located on the 'original' highway between Detroit and Chicago. Once we determined the space we needed, we went through sticker-shock from building quotes. We didn't require a real large space but ironically, a small winery license in Michigan means less than 50,000 gallons annually, so there are only a few 'large' wineries in the state. We would be in the 'very small' category if they had one (laughing). This building, which was originally a truck stop diner called Dad's Place and later a machine shop, is actually right on the way to the vineyard. It took eight months to renovate.

The tasting room bar is beautiful and has a great history.

Crick: It's made from wood that Dave Braganini gave us – coming from one of the last 12,000 gallon cypress tanks they used at the St. Julian Winery. He and Dean are old friends and most of the fruit from the Lawton Ridge Vineyard went to St. Julian. We had the wood milled down and made into the bar and we have a picture showing five or six of those cypress tanks all lined up – of course, now they're all stainless steel.

How would you describe Lawton Ridge's wine style?

Crick: We're striving to make wines that pair well with foods and wines that reflect where the fruit is grown. Michigan grapes have a tendency to be higher in acidity with less sugar but we think that makes for a well-balanced food friendly wine.

What advice would you give someone who wanted to open a winery?

Crick: A longtime Michigan winemaker, who shall remain nameless, once told us to find something else to do (laughing). Seriously, if the person is committed to making quality wine and really enjoys it, I would make sure they understand a winery is a very labor and financially intense business – there's a lot of work and equipment expense going into each bottle of wine.

You spend a lot of time in the tasting room. What is the most unusual question you've been asked?

Crick: A gentleman asked me what was the best way to store a bottle of wine once it's opened. When I asked him for how long – he said 'maybe a year.' Now, I'm not sure if he was drinking it by the teaspoon or maybe a glass every other month but a year...?

Your wine is too good to wait that long! Thanks Crick.

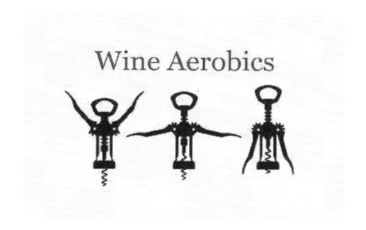

ROBINETTES APPLE HAUS & WINERY
Spies, Pies And Wine

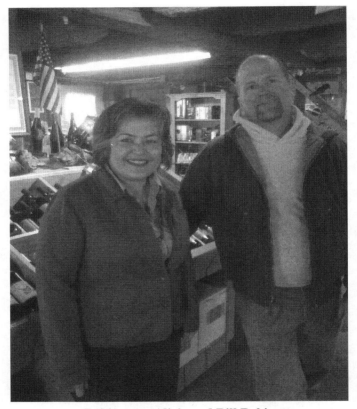

Robinette – Alicia and Bill Robinette

Just a few miles north of Grand Rapids, you can immerse yourself into the countryside of the Robinette family-owned fruit orchards. It's hard to believe you're within sight of a busy 4-lane highway. Follow the smells of the cider mill and bakery, which will take you back to the real treat – the wine cellar in the lower floor of Robinette's beautifully restored barn.

It all started when Barzilla Robinette bought the farm in 1911, which was called the Oakland Fruit Farm back then. Now the fourth generation Robinettes are operating the 125 acres located on 4-Mile Rd. west of East Beltline Hwy. "I think my husband Ed, who is the eldest son, is 'officially' the President of the business," said Manager Alicia Robinette. "We don't really make much of titles around here (laughing) – we all just dig in and do what needs to be done." And there's plenty to get done.

For more than a half-century they operated as a wholesale apple supplier and then gravitated to retail when Ed's father Jim built the cider mill in 1971. The Apple Haus came along two years later, which includes the bakery, a lunch counter and fresh fruit market. The winery was added in 2006, with Ed's brother Bill serving as the winemaker.

Alicia was raised five minutes from the farm but she met Ed in the high school band – she played clarinet and he played the trumpet. They got married and she pursued a business degree. The farm needed a manager, so after working with several other businesses she came on board. "My biggest responsibility, by far, is to make sure payroll gets out on time (laughing)." The farm usually has around 10 employees during winter hours but expands to over 100 during the fall harvest.

"Pick-your-own is fairly new for us but the winery has brought in a whole new batch of customers," Alicia said. "We currently offer 21 Michigan-made wines, with the latest additions being Royal Raspberry Spumante and Bill's Special Cider."

No doubt the customers are getting the royal treatment and finding Robinette Cellars to be a very special place.

Interview with Alicia Robinette:

Your labels all have very bright colors with a robin on them...who came up with that idea?

Alicia: Ed thought it was a good way to identify our product on the shelf and the robin helps customers remember our name. The barn was remodeled in 1985 for office space, a dining area and the gift shop. The tasting room itself is on the ground floor, which used to be the stables for the horses back when that was the mode of transportation. They were hitched to wagon to haul the fruit into Grand Rapids, which was quite a trip back in the day. It has a wine cellar feel and atmosphere so we all thought Robinette Cellars sounded right.

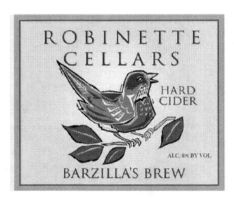

One of your wines is Barzilla's Brew and another is Bill's Special Cider. What inspired those names?

Alicia: Barzilla Robinette is Ed's great-grandfather who bought the farm in 1911. Family lore says he told everyone 'feel free NOT to name any of the children after me' and thankful no one has (laughing). But we did name our first wine after him. It's actually a biblical name. And Bill is our winemaker and we were sitting around trying to think of a name for Bill's latest creation. By consensus, we came up with Bill's Special Cider – I don't know what makes it special but it tastes good! As you can see, we don't spend a lot of time or money on market research.

It seems many of the Michigan orchards are adding a winery to their operation for another money stream. Was that the case for Robinette Cellars?

Alicia: Bill had been making ciders and wines for quite a while and there were several other fruit orchards that led the way. By comparison, we are a small operation and we are very vulnerable to Mother Nature. A good example was 2012, where it got into the 80's in March and then there was a big freeze in April. We lost all but a little of our entire fruit crop. So we are always looking for alternative income sources. The winery was a natural extension to our overall business plan. We received a lot of help from Uncle John's, Black Star and Fenn Valley wineries. It's amazing how willing some people are to lend a helping hand.

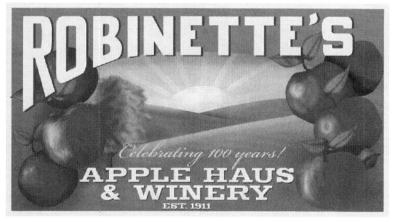

In good years, when you aren't incurring the wrath of Mother Nature, you grow a good variety of fruits. Does Bill make the choices for wines or is that by consensus as well?

Alicia: Bill makes what he likes, which is usually wines that are on the dry side. We give him input and sometimes he listens – sometimes he doesn't (laughing). Although we do have some people who prefer dry wines, most of our customers like the sweeter fruit wines. So we're always encouraging Bill to go sweeter.

I would imagine you get a very diverse demographic in your tasting room. But is there a common question that almost everyone asks?

Alicia: 'How is hard cider made?' 'How do you go from apples to fresh juice to hard cider?' And don't ask me to explain it – that's Bill's area (laughing). We do actually get requests for 5 or 10 gallons of fresh cider to take home and ferment for their own hard cider, to which I say 'go for it.' Surprisingly, a lot of people don't realize you can make wine from fruit – they think all wines are made from just grapes. But that's one of the fun things about wine. If you can get it to ferment, you can make wine from dandelions, rhubarb – I even saw someone had made wine out of tomatoes.

So many of your activities here are family-oriented. Was it difficult adding wines to your marketing strategy?

Alicia: Some people are surprised we offer wines but I've found wines to be pretty easy to market. I would imagine any alcohol-based product wouldn't be that difficult. The exception is wine sales online, which is still a hassle with all the hoops you have to go through but that's understandable.

Is there a plan to expand Robinette Cellars to retail stores in the future?

Alicia: The Cellars has been a valuable addition to the operation and I would love to see Bill get carried away with more wines. But right now it would require a new building and bigger tanks to dramatically increase production. I see it in the future but we'll take baby steps first. Unless you've got an independent money source, so many times a business that expands rapidly usually ends up in financial trouble. We obviously want to stay in business (laughing), but really, we're providing our customers with good tasting Michigan wines and we'll grow with the demand.

Just ship Mother Nature a case of Barzilla's Brew to keep her in a good mood and I'm sure Robinettes' will be around for a long time. Thanks Alicia.

> See the Robinette ad on page 413.

**Everyone has to believe in something.
I believe I'll have another glass of wine.**

SAINTS PRESERVE US AS THEY HAVE AT THE ST. JULIAN WINERY

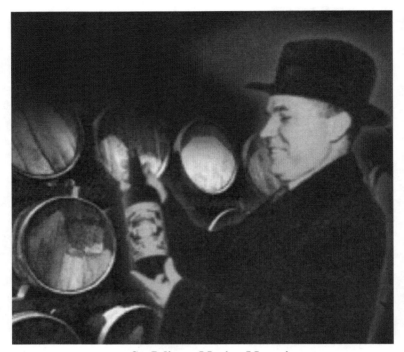

St. Julian – Marian Meconi

St. Julian Winery, named after the patron saint of founder Mariano Meconi's hometown of Faleria, Italy, continues to prosper despite multiple challenges – obviously preserved by its saint, some hard work and a little luck. As long as he can remember, the winery in Paw Paw has been a part of grandson David Braganini's life.

Now the President of St. Julian, which is the largest and oldest winery in Michigan, David takes pride in nurturing his family legacy in the wine industry. He is also striving to make the family-owned winery a beacon for the future.

"When I was growing up, all the grapes were picked by hand," David said. "We filled old beer lugs, put our tag in each one and were paid that night after the count at twenty-five cents per lug. My brother and I figured if we switched tags with others, we'd get a lot more money. The first night it worked well – the second night the migrant workers almost started a riot (laughing). Our grandfather whopped us pretty good for that stunt."

David's father, Apollo Braganini, eventually struck out on his own and the family moved to Pennsylvania in 1967, where David finished high school and got a college degree in business. Through a series of family deaths, Apollo returned to Paw Paw in 1973 to run St. Julian. Upon graduation, David returned as Director of Sales. "If my father knew at the time how poorly the company was performing, I don't think he would have come back," David said. "He never said it but I felt it. When we left Michigan in 1967, business was brisk. In the six years we were away, the market for Michigan dessert wine changed dramatically."

In 1978, David took charge of the struggling winery along with his high school friend Chas Catherman, who was the Head Winemaker. It came at a time when there were just a handful of wineries in Michigan.

Today, St. Julian has over 800 acres of grapes under contract as well as their own vineyards, an extensive product list, brandy and vodka spirits, as well as a growing bulk wine and juice business. The winery has developed the 100% Michigan Braganini Reserve line of premium single vineyard estate grown wines on their Mountain Road Vineyard as well as other select varietals from vineyards in Berrien and Van Buren counties.

Interview with David Braganini:

Reading the history of St. Julian, I can't help but marvel at the number of times the company has overcome misfortune and challenges. How bad was it when you started in 1973?

David: Surviving Prohibition was challenging enough but when my mother died in 1971, the Winery burned down during the funeral Mass and unfortunately, there was inadequate fire insurance. Less than two years later both of my uncles who were managing the place died within six weeks of each other. My grandfather had already retired and moved to Florida, so St. Julian was suddenly a ship with no captain and no maps. It was the ultimate challenge!

What turned it around?

David: Hiring my friend Chas was one of the best moves we ever made – he worked incessantly for 35 years at the company. He ran the inside and I ran the roads, while my dad was biting his fingernails (laughing). But I believed in the company – I didn't know any better I guess. In 1977, I convinced the bank to put the personal guarantee on me and by the early 80's I took control of the family-owned stock. My father foresaw the collapse of dessert wine in the early 70's and had planted substantial acres of French hybrid grapes for the production of table wines, which truly saved us. We now make two premium dessert wines and the rest are hybrid and pure Michigan vinifera table wines.

I read that you used to go to dinner at your grandfather's house every Sunday. What were those table conversations like?

David: I don't think my father could tolerate talking business at the dinner table, which my grandfather insisted on doing – I remember dad always coming up with reasons on why he had to go into the winery after dinner. When I was young they would always be drinking C K Mondavi Burgundy and I could never understand why they weren't drinking their own product – I later realized they didn't make a dry red table wine back then.

What is the biggest difference between the northern grape-growing regions and the southern Michigan regions?

David: An advantage we have here is a longer growing season by about 2 weeks or more. They are over 200 miles further north. Surprisingly, their winter temperatures don't usually dip below zero as often as ours do, probably because they are even more protected by the surrounding waters.

You have a vast collection of wine industry artifacts. What is the most unique in your collection?

David: I've got a 1928 Evenrude outboard motor that folds up into a box. Let me tell you how that relates to the wine industry. They only made them for two years and probably sold most of them to people in Detroit and Windsor. Bootleggers would load their boats up each night with "product" and shoot across the river, unbolt the motor, put it in its carrying case and leave the boat on the Detroit side. They then hitched a ride back to Canada with the motor in a briefcase. After a week or so they would tie all the empty boats together and tow them all back to Windsor and repeat the exercise.

You also have the first woman, Nancie Corum, who is a commercial winemaker. Has it been tough for her in a male dominated professional?

David: She has impeccable training and is brilliant. She deals with the growers, directs the harvest, makes the wine and writes all the cellar orders. I think she is so confident that she can accept constructive criticism and you can't say that about very many of the ego driven winemakers out there. It may have been a struggle at first but her body of work speaks for itself. I hold her in the highest esteem.

During your tenure, what would you pick as the highlights in St. Julian's history?

David: We won the Michigan Product of the Year Award for our winery in Frankenmuth in 1986. The Pope used our wine when he said Mass in the Silverdome. And I think seeing my grandfather tasting our wine in his later years and being amazed we could make a great tasting table wine – I don't think he ever thought those grapes would grow here.

St. Julian has had quite a few 'firsts' including starting up a tasting room. How did that come about?

David: The primary reason was the opening of I-94 in 1959. People started stopping in out of curiosity and my dad built a bar and started serving samples. In 1981, we established a new winery in Frankenmuth, which was and still is the #1 tourist attraction in Michigan. The law was eventually changed to allow off-site tasting rooms and the light bulb went on when I was coming back from a grand opening of our Mackinaw City store. I spotted a vacant Stuckey's Restaurant, which all have huge highway signage – at one time we operated 5 of them – great locations.

The Heron lines of wine are some of your most successful sellers. Would you share the story behind the name?

David: After my dad passed away in 1997, many times I would spot a blue heron while sitting on the dock at the lake where he lived. It almost became a good luck charm – I would see one and good things happened. I'm not into reincarnation like Shirley MacLaine but I looked at those herons as a sign from my dad. So when blue bottles became popular and we were trying to come up with a name that represented Michigan, I guess it was my dad speaking Blue Heron to us. Now, we also have Red and White Heron Wine and Grey Heron Vodka - I think he would be pleased with the results.

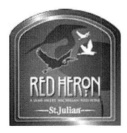 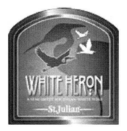 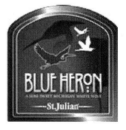

Tell us about the how and why of the Braganini Reserve wines...

David: They are truly single vineyard and estate bottled premium 100% Michigan wines. Early on in Gallo's evolution, they were making great table wines but encountered terrific resistance to the name in the marketplace. So they began to either create new and interesting brand names or bought wineries with strong brand recognition. Most people would be quite surprised at the number of wine brands that Gallo produces. It was a quest for us to break away from the St. Julian name, as well, in producing vinifera wines – like reading the fine print and finding out a Lexus is made by Toyota (laughing). We sell almost all of the Braganini Reserve through our wine club or tasting sites and a few select restaurants.

And the Braganini line also will continue with your daughter Angela, working for St. Julian. Is she the heir apparent?

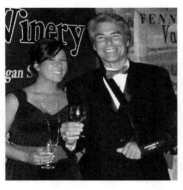

David: Angela is doing a great job here and we have a strong and experienced board of directors, which is a real asset. Although I have been here over 40 years, I don't plan on retiring anytime soon but much like my grandfather, my father and myself, she will set her own course. She studied marketing at Michigan State and has brought a fresh and creative approach to our business. I can think of no better hands in which to leave the place.

Here's to many more great years and many more great wines – thanks David.

See the St. Julian ad on page 416.

12 CORNERS WINERY
Don't Miss Your Corner

Take the last exit south on I-196 before reaching I-94 and you're almost there. Go just a few corners past the long gone hamlet of Twelve Corners, Michigan and you've reached the 12 Corners Winery. If you miss your exit, you can see it right there on the hill as you turn on 94 – but it's well worth your time to go back.

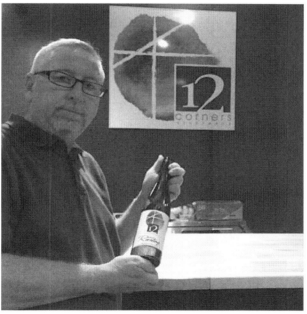

Doug Oberst was raised on a farm in Gratiot County. He went to Alma College and graduated in 1980 - when the country was about to enter an agricultural recession and farms were in trouble (remember Willie Nelson's Farm Aid Concert?). Doug spent quite a few years as an agricultural banker helping farmers stay afloat.

Then he started a consulting business advising ag-clients on handling financial matters. "In the course of my consulting work, I became aware of an emerging industry that I felt was on the verge of really taking off," Doug said. "All the signs were pointing to the winery and wine grape growing business.

His wife Gloria grew up on a vineyard/blueberry farm near Benton Harbor so they both were familiar with agricultural activities. They built a home out in the country in 2006 on property that already had grapevines. That property became the first of several farm properties that would lead to the development of a winery. "My wife really has an affinity for grapes but not so much blueberries," Doug remembered. "If I had bought a blueberry farm, the marriage may have ended quickly (laughing)."

Doug was one of three primary partners who capitalized the venture, the other two being Jim Hovinga from Grand Haven and Mark Graham from Breckenridge. Several others asked to participate, so a group was formed named "Twelve Corners Vineyards, LLC."

Concord and Niagara vines were replaced with varieties like Muscato, Cab Sauv, Riesling and Traminette. It took three years of planning and planting before the opening of a tasting room in South Haven in the fall of 2012. Then a 2,500 sq. ft. facility, just off the Red Arrow Highway, was opened in July 2013 and was called the 12 Corners Winery.

"My partners and I are all successful businessmen," Doug said. "We felt the simplest, basic principle dictated the placement of our winery – location, location, location. In today's world, people are busy and shouldn't have to search for a winery. So we have easy on – easy off accessibility and a fantastic view."

Between the two locations, they have 34 employees and currently a nineteen wine selection.

Interview with Doug Oberst:

Where does the name 12 Corners Winery come from – are there really 12 corners somewhere?

Doug: Twelve Corners is an intersection that used to be a small town just about 600 yards north of the winery. Red Arrow Hwy. (old 94) forms a triangle with two other roads that make 12 distinct separate corners. There are a couple old country churches still there but it's no longer recognized by the postal service as a town. It does still come up on Google Maps and Mapquest though.

Is your logo an artistic view of the old settlement?

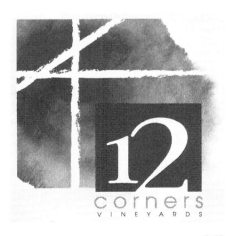

Doug: It's interesting how that evolved. I started out with a Twelve Corners wallpaper on my computer, which was the name of one of the three farms that make up the vineyard. One of my partners walked by and said 'hey, that should be the name of our winery.' We hired a marketing firm to pitch a bunch of ideas for logos but none of them really grabbed our interest. Finally, in desperation, their spokesperson said 'well, there's one more but I don't think you'll it.' It's the colorful abstract aerial view of the 12 corners – it grows on you and the public loves it.

You opened a tasting room in South Haven to get some experience. How did that work out?

Doug: We hit the ground running on the day after Thanksgiving in 2012 – no lavish grand opening – we simply unlocked the doors. It has far exceeded our expectations and we've had great cooperation from the city of South Haven. We have found the people there are primarily coming in for the wine tasting experience – a walk in crowd. The Benton Harbor facility, which we opened six months later, are people who have made a commitment to stop in – a destination point. We've found them wanting more than just the wine but also the whole vineyard experience.

Did you already have a vision of what you wanted to build?

Doug: Actually, we toured a lot of Michigan wineries and some in Napa Valley and Sonoma, California. Obviously, we wanted to emulate the successful wineries but we spent a lot of development time evaluating what we thought the people liked and tried to incorporate as many of those things as possible. From the compliments we've received, I think we got it right.

As a new winery, what have you done to get your name out there to the public?

Doug: One of the problems we ran into, which I'm assuming all new wineries have had, was not knowing when we were going to be licensed and able to open because of the governmental bureaucracy. You don't want to commit to a huge amount of marketing expenditures until you know when the business can open officially. But we've got billboards on all the major highways, done some radio advertising and have ads in the print media, especially the southwest Michigan tour guides, also the *Grand Rapids* magazine and one called *Michigan Blue*, which has a large circulation in Chicago. By all indications the people are finding us.

With 115 total acres and 30 already in vines, are there plans to expand?

Doug: We're really not sure right now. It's very capital intensive to plant grapes and quite frankly, we want to get very good at the level we're at before thinking about expanding.

Your website mentions 'wines from Michigan's famed Gold Coast.' Where is the gold coast in Michigan?

Doug: That seems to be the current buzzwords for this area, which I interpret as the sandy beaches of Lake Michigan – anywhere from the Michigan/Indiana line up to the Saugatuck/Holland area. We're just hoping there's enough gold around to include us (laughing).

How have the rest of the southwest Michigan wineries accepted 12 Corners?

Doug: We've had wonderful cooperation and assistance from neighboring wineries. You hear about competition being welcomed in the wine industry because the ultimate is reaching 'critical mass' like in the Traverse area – it then becomes a tourist destination event – taking the wine tours. Southwest Michigan is going though the same thing. But we owe a tremendous dept of gratitude to the pioneer wineries of Michigan. They cut the brush away from the road and paved the way for us.

You have a Riverstone series of wines and a Blue Creek series – how did you come up with those?

Doug: My daughter came up with the Riverstone name and Blue Creek is very near the winery and again, is a tribute to the local area. The reality is there are no books or internet website services you can research to get names for all the wines – and, it's on going, continually evolving. So you end up going to all your wine drinking friends and relatives and asking for names. We took it a step further and added an incentive – a covenant with the people - if we use your idea, you get a free case of wine!

I'm thinking of names already – thanks, Doug.

See the 12 Corners ad on page 392.

WHITE PINE WINERY
Doctor Dave Knows His Wines

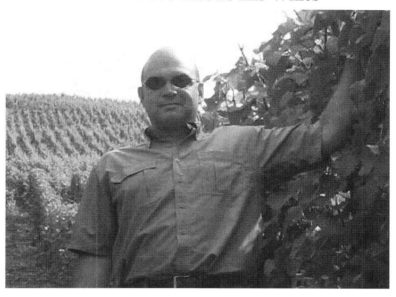

Dave Miller came to Michigan in 1983 to work on a masters degree in viticulture at Michigan State University. He left twelve years later with a PhD that led to a job at the oldest winery in the state and eventually his own winery.

While pursuing his degrees, Dave took a job working as a technician running the grape & wine research program for Dr. Stan Howell at MSU. Along the way, he met a local girl from Lansing named Sandy, who would become Mrs. Miller.

"After getting my masters degree, I started looking for work in the wine industry," Dave recalled. "When I applied for a job at a California winery I was told if I didn't have a degree from the University of California at Davis or Fresno, work out there wasn't going to happen. I guess they didn't know the chairman of the UC Davis viticulture program for years was one of Dr. Howell's graduates."

"I decided to seek my fame and fortune in the world of academics," Dave chuckled. "I went on to get my doctorate and then took a job as a winemaker for St. Julian Winery."

He immediately began training the grape growers in proper cropping and canopy management and focusing their attention on improving the quality of grapes supplied to St. Julian. Under his tutelage, the winery sales increased significantly and he began the Braganini Reserve line of premium wines. "I was given the latitude to develop many new wines and I also helped get their distilled spirits program off the ground."

After thirteen years, Dave reached a point in his career where he was thinking 'now what?' "St. Julian's offered me an opportunity to put my viticulture training to practical use," he said. "But by 2009 I was searching for the next big challenge."

That challenge became the White Pine Winery. With a goal of creating a vineyard and winery that produced a higher end wine for the more sophisticated palate, Dave and Sandy opened White Pine in 2010. They located their tasting room in downtown St. Joseph and feature a selection of fifteen wines.

Nearly in sight of beautiful sand dunes and close enough to feel the breezes from Lake Michigan, the White Pine Winery is a great setting to try some of Dr. Dave's great wine.

Interview with Dave Miller:

During your academic research, did you develop a wine grape growing philosophy?

Dave: I learned you have to grow grapes that are suited to the local environment. Michigan wine grape growers are beginning to focus on that. California tried to import vineyard management techniques that worked in France but failed in California. By the same token, we have to apply a management approach that is consistent with our vine/environment interaction to produce the best wines.

You mentioned the California viticulture programs – how is the MSU program viewed in the wine world?

Dave: Stan Howell's program was respected around the wine world. During my doctoral years, we had winemakers from around the world come to learn about what we were doing.

Your PhD focused on crop levels in growing grapes. In layman's terms, why is that important?

Dave: If the wine grapes aren't at the proper crop levels, they will lack in flavor, color and varietal characters. Just because you can get high yields and still keep the sugar level high (around 20 brix) doesn't mean it will be quality wine – there are a lot of other subtle nuances happening. I worked primarily on the limits of yield based on leaf area and the length of the growing season. And that's what we deal with in Michigan – variable growing seasons.

You are known as 'Doctor Dave', which would imply you've got an unpronounceable last name...but it's Miller. So where does the Dr. Dave come from?

Dave: It started at St. Julian, whose president is Dave Braganini. He was Big Dave and I was Dr. Dave. When we opened White Pine Winery, we had an employee named Dave, so I was Dr. Dave and he was P.A. for physician's assistant.

Tell us about Sophie's Vineyard.

Dave: We planted a vineyard on our property in 1999, which was the same year our daughter Sophie was born. I loved the idea of naming the vineyard after one of the women in our family – it seemed appropriate.

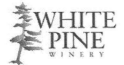 **Where does the name White Pine Winery come from?**

Dave: Michigan's state tree is the white pine. So we wanted to send a subliminal message out to the world that we're all about Michigan. Of course, we have such spectacular sand dunes around here, one of my friends suggested we do a takeoff on the old Cat Stevens song Moon Shadow and call the winery Dune Shadow. I nixed that for the winery but said we could certainly give one of our wines that name. And that's where Dune Shadow Red comes from.

You also have Red & White Expression and Serendipity…

Dave: Red and White Expression are expressions of the local soils and climate – *'terroir'* if you will. And at some point we were encountering a problem that later became a blessing and we both thought it was a serendipitous happening. So our next wine became Serendipity.

Your have a very simple but 'stately' logo on your labels. Who designed it?

Dave: My sister-in-law actually designed the label logo, which is a lone white pine hanging out over one of the Great Lakes – a great Michigan scene. She did a rough sketch and we sent it to an artist. We wanted an identifiable logo, like the Nike swoosh or the McDonalds M, someday…

The tasting room is in downtown St. Joseph. Why did you choose that location and tell us the history of your building?

Dave: I was out in Healdsburg, California, which is in Sonoma County about fifteen years ago and they had four winery tasting rooms right in the downtown area – now there are about thirty! But I always thought that was cool – you can shop, have lunch, taste some wine and walk back to your hotel room without having to drive anywhere. That's exactly what we have in downtown St. Joseph. We've got space in one of the oldest buildings downtown – it used to be a bakery, with the old pressed tin ceiling and exposed brick. We're always getting compliments on the setting and location.

And you haven't totally given up on making a fortune in academics…you're still on the faculty at MSU.

Dave: I'm an assistant professor in the Food Services Department. I teach winemaking. I still love interacting and sharing with the students. We have to teach the next generation.

Thanks for educating and sharing with us, Professor.

SOUTHEAST

BLUE WATER & OLD TOWN HALL...............273
BURGDORFS...280
CHERRY CREEK..285
GREEN BARN...294
LONE OAK..299
PENTAMERE..304
SAND HILL CRANE..................................310
SANDY SHORE..315
UNCLE JOHN'S..320

**It doesn't mater is the glass is half empty or half full.
There is clearly room for more wine.**

BLUE WATER WINERY AND VINEYARDS
OLD TOWN HALL WINERY
Think Globally, Drink Locally

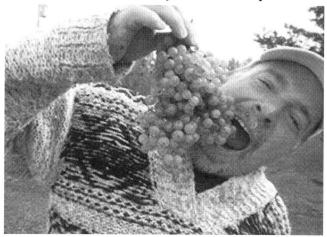

How do two computer software executives from Chicago end up making wine in the thumb area of Michigan? It makes sense once you've been to the Blue Water Vineyards and the Old Town Hall Winery and of course, you try their wines.

Connie Currie and Steve Velloff met while working in the world of computers in Boston. They eventually gravitated to Chicago and started their own software company dealing with 'intellectual properties' in 1994.

Connie was raised in southeast Michigan and Steve grew up just outside of St. Louis, MO. "As a software executive, you do a lot of wining and dining," Steve recalled. "My grandfather actually grew up on a vineyard in Europe and I come from a family of home winemakers. Connie and I eventually got tired of the big city and I got tired of having no place to walk the dogs, so Michigan was the logical choice to be close to Connie's family."

Having worked with a few startup companies, they knew how much energy it takes to get a new venture off the ground but their love of animals and wine drew them to farmland. The east side of Michigan is an agricultural haven with a huge body of water called Lake Huron close by, so they started researching winemaking and suitable land for a vineyard.

They took MSU extension courses and went through the University of California at Davis viticulture certification program. "It's a different kind of physical labor working in a vineyard all day but sitting at a computer for fourteen hours straight can be taxing too," Steve chuckled.

He and Connie purchased 30 acres just south of Port Sanilac and planted three acres of Cab Franc, Pinot Noir and Chardonnay wine grapes in 2005. They have added additional acreage each year and opened the Blue Water Vineyards and Winery in 2009.

As the business grew, they bought a building in Lexington just seven miles south of the vineyards and opened the Old Town Hall Winery in 2011. "When working with intellectual properties the satisfaction is in the end result and then it's gone," Steve said. "With wine, you plant the vines, work the vineyard, make the wine and you actually can see your customer enjoy and appreciate the results. It's a whole different kind of satisfaction."

Interview with Steve Velloff:

What is the history of the farm you purchased in Sanilac County?

Steve: It was known as the Holverson Farm, with the original 4-room farmhouse built in the 1850's. An addition was built on in 1886, right after the huge fire that swept across eastern Michigan and burned over 1 million acres. The farm was probably the usual 640 acres but has been divided many times - we have 30 acres. It stayed in the Halverson family until the 1950's and most owners since have used the property as a hunting retreat.

There are very few grape growers in eastern Michigan that left a good growing record for you to research. What varietals have thrived under your care?

Steve: Actually, the Cabernet Franc, Pinot Noir and Chardonnay have all thrived. We recently increased our Cab Franc acreage and that wine won us a gold medal in the San Francisco International Wine Contest in July 2013.

From your initial research until now, you have eight years of vineyard growth - are you getting the 'lake effect' to protect your vines?

Steve: The simple answer is yes. What makes our property unique is the last glacier that formed Lake Huron actually created somewhat of a geographic bowl for us. The result is we stay a little cooler in the spring, which causes the grapes to wake up slower and we stay warmer longer into the fall, which helps the grapes get riper.

Your label features your wine dogs Bernie and Goldie...and you do something called the Harvest for the Hounds. Tell us about that.

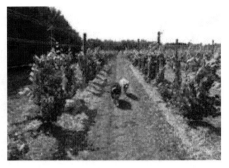

Steve: Connie was snapping pictures in the vineyard and took one of our two pals walking down through a row of Chardonnay. We both thought it was a cool picture. Bernie, we think, is an Australian Shepard who we rescued from the Humane Society in Chicago. Goldie was a stray on the streets - she adopted us. We use the Harvest for the Hounds as a fundraiser for the local Humane Society. What can I say, we love animals.

What was the origin of your Blessing of the Vines?

Steve: In 2012, a tour bus from Grosse Pointe was coming through Lexington on their way to Port Sanilac. Connie was talking to one of our customers about it – they were looking for another activity to do in the area and mentioned Father Mark Haydu from the Vatican was with the tour. So Connie suggested they come out to Blue Water and have the Father bless the vineyard. Everyone had a great time and it looks like we're going to make it an annual event now.

I read that you won another gold medal in San Francisco with something called Norton Red – what's the story behind that?

Steve: The Norton grape is the state grape of Missouri. When I visit my parents in the St. Louis area, I like to go visit some of the wineries. There's a little town called Grafton – no stoplight and maybe 600 people but they have four wineries and five micro-breweries in town. I sourced the Norton grapes from there. It's a native American grape that requires a long growing season, which we don't have but I tweaked it and came up with Norton Red – it tastes earthy, like a Malbec. To send two dry reds out to California and have them judged as gold medal recipients says a lot for Michigan's quality of wines. It was great publicity for Sanilac County as well.

Do you have a winemaking philosophy?

Steve: We try to do two things – first, we try to make wines we like to drink but we also listen to our customers. So, second, we adjust to what they say to round out our wine offerings. We know people have differing palates so we make every effort not to influence their wine tastes toward our preferences. The idea is to match their tastes with a wine that suits them. Between Blue Water and the Old Town Hall Winery we offer a lot of choices.

OLD TOWN HALL WINERY

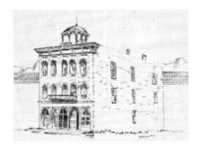

Tell us about purchasing the Old Town Hall.

Steve: We were in a build or buy expansion mode at Blue Water. It's popular for Michigan wineries to expand by having a tasting room nearer to the populated/high traffic areas. The Masons built the Town Hall (it wasn't old then) in 1876. Initially, it was a fire hall and had offices on the first floor, the second floor was an opera house and the third floor was the Masonic Temple. The Village of Lexington decided to build a new facility back in the 1980's. The building then was converted into a hardware store and pharmacy. When those owners moved out, the building was vacant for about five years before we purchased and renovated it into a tasting room, bottling and oak aging facility.

How does the wine selection at Old Town Hall differ from Blue Water?

Steve: We offer the Blue Water wine selection, which is all estate grown, at both locations but The Old Town Hall Winery wines are sourced grapes like the Norton or various fruits. We also opened the Lexington micro-brewery there in 2013.

The building is perfect for holding events. What have you had there?

Steve: The Blue Water Film Festival has come in for a fundraiser, showing a few film shorts. We also host one of the stages for the Thumbfest Music Festival in town – we have an 'open mic' there once a month. We're really open to any form of entertainment that'll be fun and bring in a crowd.

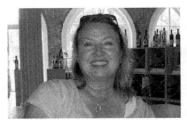

How do yours and Connie's palates differ?

Steve: Connie has a really good feel for tannin structure and the sensations associated with wine when you're drinking it. For instance, she can detect when a wine is too tannic or has too much alcohol. She has a good nose for aromas. I have a better ability to detect sweetness. We complement each other well during our tasting trials.

Where does your customer base come from?

Steve: We have a strong local base – our wines are currently in four or five local restaurants. The weekend crowd is coming from Wayne, Oakland and Macomb counties. We actually are getting quite a few visitors from Ontario, Canada as well.

The name Old Town Hall is very obvious but why Blue Water?

Steve: This is known as the 'Blue Water Area' and of course, the bridge between Port Huron and Sarnia is called the Blue Water Bridge. Originally, we were called the Adagio Estates – adagio is a musical term meaning a slow leisurely dance. But people thought it was a family name or a cheese or something (laughing). So we decided to change the name to something regionally specific.

We'll leisurely sip the wines at Blue Water and then make our way down to Lexington for some dancing at the Old Town Hall – thanks Steve.

WINE COUNTRY IN HASLETT?
BURGDORF'S WINERY MAKES IT SO!

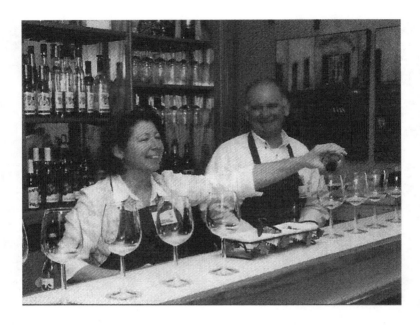

If you look east of US 127, north of I-96 and south of I-69 on a map, you'll find the town of Haslett, Michigan, which is noted for being...well, east of Lansing. When more wine drinkers realize there are wineries in Michigan producing great tasting wine and NOT in the northwest or southwest grape growing regions of the state, they will discover Haslett is also the home of Burgdorf's Winery.

Dave Burgdorf grew up on a self-sustaining farm in west central Illinois and became a vegetation specialist for the United States Dept. of Agriculture. His future bride, Deb, was from Chicago and became a forestry/fermentation microbiologist. They met in college and their two worlds became one, with wine following shortly thereafter.

"Our family farm had a big patch of wild black raspberries on it," recalled Dave. "When Deb finally said 'STOP – I can only make so much jelly, cobbler and pies' I said let's make some wine. I'll admit it was god-awful tasting stuff. It made your cheeks red and your toes numb. But we mixed it with a little 7-Up and drank it anyway (laughing)."

Fast-forward through 35 years of winemaking and 33 years of marriage...jobs brought the Burdorfs to mid-Michigan and the spark to build a winery started in 2001. Eventually, their dream came to fruition with the opening of Burgdorf's Winery in 2005 and they improved dramatically on their winemaking skills.

It took some time, but their persistence paid off when they tweaked those wild black raspberries all the way to Perfection, which is one of their best selling wines.

Interview with Dave and Deb Burgdorf:

Your winery name is also your last name. Was that a tough choice?

Deb: It sounded right and we didn't feel intimidated by using it. So far – so good.

Dave: It's personal and it's who we are. We make all of our own wines. It's our creations using our expertise.

How do you decide the names of your wines?

Dave: Many times if it's something other than the grape name (pinot noir, syrah, chardonnay, etc.), we will name the wines after a place or person – we have a red named Marquette and one named Faye (first grandchild). We either grow or purchase 100% Michigan fruit from farmers who meet our specifications.

Deb: There is a blueberry wine we call A Maize N Blue and Spartan white and a sweet Vidal Blanc called Golden Temptation. If it's a blend, we try to come up with a catchy name that represents a characteristic of the wine.

I see you use mostly synthetic cork for your closure. Is there a big price difference between synthetic and real cork?

Dave: There isn't a big difference in price. Real cork comes from the cork tree, which grows primarily around the Mediterranean and Portugal. The cork itself is harvested from the bark of the tree. We actually tried to grow cork here in the United States but the conditions weren't right to allow the bark to get thick enough.

Deb: Real cork has storage issues. Bottles need to be stored on their side and if the cork doesn't stay moist and dries out, there is shrinkage, which allows air to reach the wine. I feel safer using synthetic cork, which eliminates that problem but good, bad, or better, there are very subtle differences.

When deciding what wine to make, what factors do you consider?

Dave: We listen to our customer's input and how the market is reacting to different wines. But we are a fledgling winery and come from a homemade wine background. So the creative factor really drives our wine production.

Deb: We are trying to break away from traditional fruit wines. Sometimes the customers will shy away saying 'I don't drink fruit wines' but once they try them, you can see the change on their faces. Our goal is to carve a niche and be different with the best wines we can produce.

How do you overcome a customer's preconceived opinions on fruit wines?

Dave: Let's say a customer says 'I like Merlots.' I tell 'em not to think all Merlots taste alike. Don't be disappointed if the next Merlot they try doesn't taste like the last one they tried and liked. Each winemaker should tweak their wines to make them different and hopefully as good or better than other winemakers. Don't judge a wine by just smelling it and don't judge it from just one sip – it takes about 3 or 4 sips to get all those factors in tune. Collectively, they add up to a moment in wine.

So how do a farmer and biologist end up making fruit wines in Haslett?

Deb: I have no idea (laughing). Early in my career, I found myself wading through swamps doing environmental surveys and really didn't like that. Dave was always eager to get his hands dirty. But, as he said, we've always been in that group of 'crazy' people who make wine in their basement. It was our neighbor who encouraged us to turn this hobby into a business.
Dave: We both took a serious look at what we were going to do as we approached retirement. I've always been active outdoors

but I don't play golf or fish every much. This became a great option to keep us active and creative. She's still the brains of the fermentation process, only this smells a lot better (laughing). And I still get my hands dirty.

Haslett definitely is not in a traditional winery area in Michigan. That makes you unique already but how do you make the experience unique for your customers?

Deb: When we first started, our customers kept reinforcing the idea of supporting Michigan – grown and made in Michigan. But there aren't those rolling hills covered in grapevines around here. We have a small vineyard but our tour concentrates on the whole process from the ground to the bottle. They get to see the lab, which a lot of wineries don't have and we explain the chemistry behind turning the fruit into wine.

Dave: We looked at our situation as a way of continuing to support Michigan agriculture without owning a lot of acreage ourselves. This is an opportunity to educate our customers about Michigan's natural resources and because we are a small operation, they get an up close experience. They hear our story and understand we aren't just employees – we are the winery and they are part of our journey.

And the journey to Haslett is worth taking, thanks to the Burgdorfs.

See the Burgdorf ads on the inside front cover and page 397.

CHERRY CREEK WINERY
Don't Be Fooled By The Name

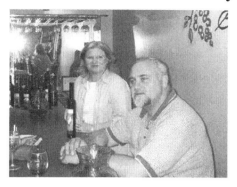

Don't look for Cherry Creek to find Cherry Creek Winery on a Michigan map. There is one location in Parma and another on U.S. 12 near Brooklyn. John and Denise Burtka now have a new winery called the Grand River Winery, which happens to be on the longest river in Michigan (more on that later!).

When John spotted Denise at a church conference, he told his Deacon 'that's the girl I'm gonna marry.' "The Deacon did mention to John that his girlfriend at the time was sitting next to him," laughed Denise. Six weeks later, they were engaged and six months later they were married – that was twenty-nine years ago.

John went on to a very successful career in the automotive supply business and Denise was a stay-at-home mom and a dental hygienist. John's wine education came from his family, wining and dining clients and multiple trips to Europe.

His skills producing homemade wine were evident when he was a regular Gold Medal and Best of Class winner in the amateur division at the Michigan State Fair. As the automotive industry started downsizing, the Burtka entrepreneurial spirit took over.

In 2002, they purchased 20 acres just off I-94 in Parma, planted vines and opened Cherry Creek Winery. In 2006, they bought the Old Schoolhouse on U.S. 12 just two miles west of Michigan International Speedway in Brooklyn; in 2010, they opened the Sleeping Bear Winery across the road from their Cherry Creek site in Parma and then opened the Grand River Winery in Jackson in 2013.

Each winery has its own personality, its own atmosphere and the Burtka flare for good wine and lots of entertainment.

Interview with Denise Burtka:

Your first winery was in Parma. Is there a Cherry Creek nearby that shares the name?

Denise: (laughing) There is no Cherry Creek! Originally we wanted our first winery to be Veritas Vineyards – vino veritas, which means 'in wine there is truth' – it has something to do with drinking wine bringing out the truth. But just a few months before opening we got word from a winery in Virginia that didn't want us to use that name because theirs was similar. Our lawyer said we could win it but would probably delay our opening by a year or so. We thought of so many different names and eventually we got suggestions from a local newspaper contest and we settled on Cherry Creek.

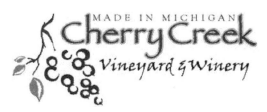

Your next winery was Sleeping Bear - where did that originate?

Denise: John always wanted to be up there near the Sleeping Bear Sand Dunes area so we trademarked that name along time ago. We just kept growing here until it just wasn't practical to expand up there. When we leased the old St. Julian tasting site in Parma, we just used that name and it's been very well received.

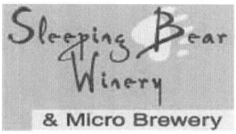

Your new place is called the Grand River Winery - was that name already there or is that something that you created?

Denise: Actually the whole place is called the Grand River Market Place and inside is the Grand River Winery, the Grand River Microbrewery, the Grand River Deli and a retail store and it's all on the Grand River (laughing). For those people that are familiar with the Jackson downtown area it used to be called Kuhl's Belltower and we've turned the parking lot into an entertainment venue every Friday night and with an event called Party on the Grand.

Which winery best fits John's personality?

Denise: It's interesting, when we first started John's desire was to make just dry red wines but that really wasn't very practical.

When we added Sleeping Bear that was our whimsical winery but here at the schoolhouse we have a lot of fun but it's also where the serious winemaking is done. So I think this place fits his personality - he likes a good time but he takes his winemaking seriously.

Tell me about your support of the arts with fundraisers and events and having artists paint your labels.

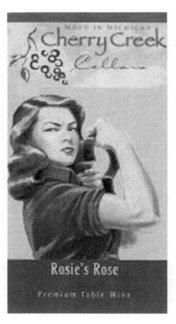

Denise: John called a friend who is a graphic artist and said he wanted original artwork on all the labels, so that's how it got started. It's more expensive but people love the idea. For example, we've got a sweet Rosé with a picture of Rosie the Riveter on the label. People buy it just because of the picture - they come back and buy another bottle because it's good wine (laughing). Neither John nor I are very artistic but at least we have always encouraged our kids to play instruments and take a foreign language.

You have the new Lynn Aleksandr reserve wines - where did that name come from?

Denise: Our daughter's name is Jessica Lynn and our son is John Aleksandr. I wish we would've thought of that 10 years ago. Jessica is at Hope College and wants to be a teacher. Johnny is in

France at a seminary - those French lessons are paying off (laughing).

You mentioned having entertainment events and you're close to Michigan International Speedway - does that help your wine sales?

Denise: Michigan International Speedway has two races a year, which are crazy weekends. Roger Curtis, the president of MIS, and John are good friends. They worked together on developing the Michigan Wine and Beer Fest every May at MIS, which has turned into a huge success. We have bands here almost every weekend and it has been a great draw - it's not unusual to get 300 to 600 people here.

Are you done expanding?

Denise: It's funny – I'm not a risk taker. I just wanted to marry a guy with a good stable job and be a mom...and my husband got us into the wine business (laughing).

We're glad he did! Thanks Denise.

AROUND THE WORLD OF WINE
BLAKE KOWNACKI, WINEMAKER AT CHERRY CREEK

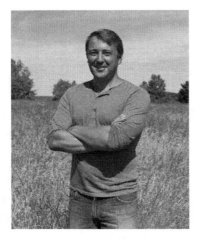

A Michigan native, Blake has traveled the world to get his hands dirty in the grapevines. From California to Australia to Brooklyn (Michigan), he's come full circle in the pursuit of making fine wines.

First, he headed west to become an organic farmer in California – growing apples, seasonal crops, lettuce and non-wine table grapes. "We were practically surrounded by vineyards and all my friends were winemakers – I was the lettuce guy," laughed Blake.

The transition to the world of wine came when he became Assistant Winemaker to Scott Hawley at Torrin Vineyards in Paso Robles, CA. "Scott is a true artisan and minimalist winemaker," Blake said. "I learned how wine is made without adding what I call the 'snake oils' of the industry to make each vintage taste the same."

From there Blake moved to Australia for a chance to work with Phillip Shaw, one of the premier winemakers down under. Eventually, the yearning to come home pulled him back to his roots in Michigan.

After reading an article about John Burtka's transition from the automotive industry to agriculture, a 'meeting of the minds' led to a job helping John create the Lynn Aleksandr Reserve line of fine wines for Cherry Creek Winery. "We're working to take Michigan wines, especially dry reds to the next level," said Blake.

The response from wine enthusiasts has indicated they are well on their way.

Interview with Blake Kownacki, winemaker at Cherry Creek Winery:

With your experience in California and Australia, you've encountered the screw cap phenomenon before it hit the Michigan wine industry – tell us your thoughts.

Blake: The whole industry is driven toward 'drink now' as opposed to actually cellaring a wine. There are very few people who put a bottle away for a long time and store it properly. With the screw cap, you are time sealing that wine and most likely drinking it shortly after purchase. In Australia, you'll see $40-$60 bottles with screw caps. Here in America, we're still stuck with the romanticism of the cork. If I'm making a red wine that is meant for aging, then 100% cork makes sense, otherwise, the screw cap is much more practical.

Cork does allow a bit of oxygen into the bottle in the aging process, correct?

Blake: Yes, the cork is porous and that allows micro-oxygenation. It's what creates the magic especially with the tannins that are binding up. You get a long molecular chain of tannins that binds with a protein in your saliva, which gives you that dry sensation. That's why there is such a wonderful interplay with a good cut of steak. The fats in the meat are mixing with the tannins and you get this fantastic flavor. As the wine ages, those chains of tannins get longer, mellow out and you get a smooth tasting wine.

But can't you keep a bottle too long, even if stored properly?

Blake: What happens over time is the tannin chains get so long they precipitate out of the solution and you lose them. That's why most 40-year-old bottles still taste good but they're probably past their prime.

Is there a rule of thumb for peak time?

Blake: It depends on the quality of fruit and region. In Michigan I don't usually get as much tannin as I'd like so peak would be about seven years. In California it would be about 12 years. The quality changes from season to season, which in turn has an effect on the aging potential. The age of the barrel has an effect as well. But all white wines should be drunk immediately with the exception of Chardonnay, which is oak aged for a year or two.

Is it just quality that creates such a wide range of pricing in wines?

Blake: There are many factors but primarily you have to include quantity as well. There is a big difference between a manufactured, mass-produced wine that has consistency in tasting exactly the same year after year and a wine that reflects the subtle differences season to season. The average wine drinker doesn't care, but a wine enthusiast looks for those nuances.

Tell us about your Detroit Project?

Blake: John Burtka was working on getting some grapevines planted on Belle Isle and turning the old casino into a winery but that's been put on hold. I am bypassing the political minefield and going directly to neighborhoods to have small plots converted into many vineyards. I hear all the time that grapes can't grow in Detroit but the reality is there are plenty of green areas and a treasure trove of marketing possibilities.

Thanks for you insights, Blake.

THE GREEN BARN
Wine In The Front – Horses In The Back

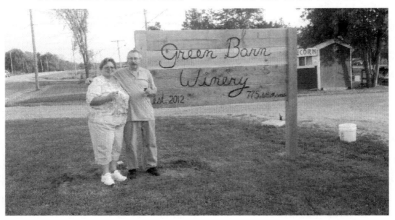

Mike and Becky Wrubel love horses and have had them for 20 years. The green barn was built in 2004 to accommodate a boarding business with a retail store in the front. They also love to make wine. The horses are still in the back but now the front accommodates a thriving winery known as the Green Barn Winery – the best of both worlds.

"We've still got plenty of room for the horses despite carving out 10 acres for fruit trees and grape vines," Becky said. "We've also got a consistent supple of fertilizer (laughing)."

They started making wine in 1981. "Actually, we attempted our first batch on our honeymoon," she said. "It didn't survive but the marriage did. My stubborn Polish husband said 'we're gonna get this right' and after blowing up some more batches, we started getting pretty good at it."

The beauty of making wine is there are no hard and fast rules. The ability to create an enjoyable wine makes it an art. The Wrubels love to blend and experiment – always willing to try new ideas. "We don't want to compete against long established wineries who make traditional vinifera wines," Becky noted. "We get all our fruit locally whenever possible and our customers love sweet wines, so we give them what they want."

They aren't beyond 'living on the edge' with their winemaking. "Mike got a supply of honey from a neighbor so he wanted to try making some mead wine. I was sitting in the office making labels and heard a raucous noise in the back. The next thing I know, his standing over me and saying 'ya wanna lick up my mess?' I looked up and he's covered in honey - he did smell pretty good (laughing)."

Plans are for Becky to retire from her job with the Macomb Intermediate School District in two years and Mike to follow in another few years from his job with the Marysville Schools. Their mishaps haven't deterred them from plans to expand into more of the barn area and go to larger tanks.

"She handles the front end – I handle the back and we meet in the middle to check for an assessment on what else needs to get done," Mike said. "Sometimes we actually work together on both ends (laughing)."

They opened in August 2012 with a dozen wines and have already expanded their wine list considerably - business is good.

Interview with Becky Wrubel:

Despite the early 'troublesome' batches, you're tasting room is loaded with a good variety of wines. Did you have any mentors?

Becky: No, actually that was one of the big disappointments early on – we didn't get much cooperation from family and friends. But we kept going by trial and error. Because of that, we've opened our doors to new winemakers and allowed them access to our knowledge and facility. We'll work with them through the fermentation process and hopefully NOT blow up any more batches (laughing).

Although you are very new, what wine would you consider one of your early successes?

Becky: We can't keep the elderberry wine on the shelf. The first week we were open it sold out. And just this week we sampled our new strawberry/rhubarb wine – it tastes just like a pie. I'm excited about that one. We have seasonal wines as well. Over the next few years, we'll adjust the wine selection to accommodate the customer's tastes.

Did you run into any major obstacles in opening the winery?

Becky: Actually the easiest part of the whole process was working with the federal government. The State was much more difficult and the Township was a challenge but I had an ace up my sleeve with them. You see, I'm also a Township Trustee and I know where most of the skeletons are (laughing). Of course, we're the first winery in this township so that alone creates some problems. I remember standing in front of the Planning Committee and asking the seven members if any of them had ever been to a winery – when I got no response I said 'see, I knew none of you know what you're talking about...now, this is the way it is.' After that we didn't have much trouble.

Your name is obvious because you are actually in a green barn. Was that your first choice?

Becky: It was our only choice. When the barn was built ten years ago we incorporated. It's simple and also amazing how quickly people have identified with it – I hear quite often 'oh, I know right where the green barn is.'

You've utilized the green barn on your labels as well. Was that planned?

Becky: We didn't at first – but we've since put everything on the computer and standardized the label. We may tweak it but we like the ones we're using now – and they're legal (laughing).

One of the wineries in Michigan is Cherry Creek but I've learned there actually isn't a Cherry Creek near by. You've got a Smiths Creek address – is there a real Smiths Creek?

Becky: Yes, there really is a Smiths Creek, but the town and area is primarily known for its dump. So we won't be using that name on any of our wines.

What is the most frequent question you get asked in the tasting room?

Becky: Quite often I'll get asked which one of our wines I like best. I always say 'which ever one is in the glass at the time.' We went to a seminar recently and one of the speakers was talking about getting a 'snob' in the tasting room critiquing the wine. We were told to just say 'doesn't that wine give you a nice dip in the back of your palate' and we were warned not to burst out laughing when they agree because there IS no dip back there!

I did try your wine and didn't feel a dip at all…thanks Becky.

See the Green Barn ad on page 406.

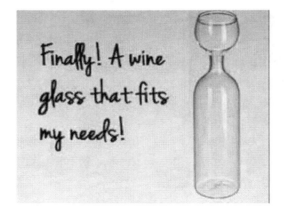

LONE OAK VINEYARD ESTATE
Taking The High Ground

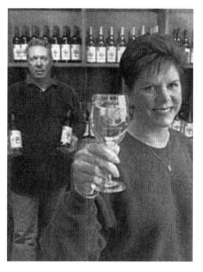

If you traveled the same latitude approximately 4,000 miles due east of Grass Lake, Michigan you'd be on the border of France and Spain, arguably two of the best wine regions in the world. Considering Lone Oak Vineyard Estate sits on that latitude and is one of the elevation highpoints of southeast Michigan (1100 ft.), it makes perfect sense why Kip and Dennise Barber thought French and German grape varieties would grow there. So when someone asks 'do grapes grow in Grass Lake?' Answer yes, and they're producing great tasting wines too.

The Barbers met on a blind date back in 1990 and it was Dennise who introduced Kip to great white wine. "The light bulb went on and I started realizing the difference between cheap wines and the good stuff," laughed Kip.

Admitting he has an obsessive personality, Kip, a Ferndale native, bought a winemaking book and made 35 bottles of white wine from one vine he planted in his backyard. The next year, he planted his ENTIRE backyard in vines.
He was a woodworking antique restorer and Dennise was a flight attendant. In their spare time, they began traveling the United

States visiting wineries. They married in 1995 and by then, Kip was 'a full-blown wine junkie.' Initially, a plan was developed to combine savings in a 'dream-home' account but after many late night discussions and negotiations, the account name changed to 'dream winery' account.

They found a hilly, forested 25-acre plot between Ann Arbor and Jackson, just south of I-94 in Grass Lake. "I realized a majority of the trees would have to be cleared to build the vineyard but I just knew I couldn't cut this one huge, majestic oak tree down," Kip said. "So Dennise said 'then let's call it the Lone Oak Vineyard' and that was it."

They moved from Ferndale in 1997 to their Jackson County property and eventually cleared 24 acres to plant classic European wine grape varieties. The tasting room opened in 2002 and Lone Oak Vineyard Estate wines can be found in a multitude of retail locations in southern Michigan.

Interview with Kip and Dennise Barber:

Was there really only one lone oak on the Lone Oak Vineyard Estate property?

Kip: No, actually, it was nearly all oaks but "our" tree was the biggest. Dennise and I hugged the tree trunk and our hands couldn't touch. Eventually, the new tasting room will be built out of the oaks we took down and be right into the hillside behind that signature tree.
Dennise: The other interesting fact we noticed about the new name was the initials spell out L.O.V.E., which has become our slogan – you're going to LOVE it at Lone Oak Vineyard Estate.

How did you develop the label design?

Kip: Dennise has an artist friend who looked at the property and came up with several 'concept' drawings. We picked what we liked from each along with the font for the writing. I wanted something simple but elegant. It was a collaborative effort and I think we nailed it.

You have some very clever names for your wines – who gets to pick those?

Kip: Our traditional wines are recognized by the name of the grape, which are French and German varieties. Some of the blends and specialty wines we collaborate on the name choice. Vin du Roi, which means 'Wine of the King', is a bold red blend. Empty Nester is a white blend that speaks 'the kids are gone, now it's your time to relax.' Puppy Love is a sweet, fun Rosé.

Dennise: We are sticking with the L.O.V.E. theme with names like Honeymoon Sweet, Love's First Blush, or French Kiss – different phases of love at different times in your life. We've had a lot of fun with it and our customers have gotten a kick out of it as well.

Speaking of Puppy Love, I understand your wine dog Ozzy is quite famous. Tell us about that.

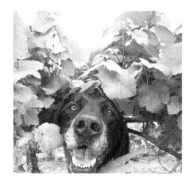

Kip: Our black lab Ozzy was on the cover of the book *Wine Dogs USA* and so we released Puppy Love at the same time.

Dennise: We had a special book-signing weekend with Ozzy putting his paw print on the books…pawtographed copies.

When your obsession started, did you have someone 'show you the ropes' so to speak, or did you just venture out on your own?

Kip: That's interesting because we traveled to many different wineries and starting out, I couldn't stand red wine. While in California, I bought a bunch of cheap wine at Trader Joe's – whites and reds. While I was being chauffeured from winery to winery, I started drinking some of the reds and I was getting a little 'baked' but I also started loving those reds! I started really listening and was really starting to understand – well, at least I thought I understood. So really, I've never sought advice. I've always been on a self-guided tour, more or less (laughing).

As a self-taught winemaker, what was the biggest obstacle to overcome?

Kip: How to grow quality grapes. There's an old saying – 'you can make bad wine from good grapes but you can't make good wine from bad grapes' and it is SO true.

Did you have a goal in mind when your dream fund changed to a winery?

Kip: When we were touring wineries, I was buying $20 to $30 bottles of wine and after drinking them, I kept thinking most weren't worth the money they cost. So my first ambition was to eventually produce a good wine that was worth its price and could stand next to any comparably priced wine in the world.

So is that your mindset when pricing Lone Oak wines?
Kip: To me, it's not about the all-mighty dollar. Is Dennise cringing (laughing)? I wanted to price my wines so the customer sees value and will brag about them to their friends.

Your wine list features estate grown reds – Merlot, Pinot Noir and Cabernet Sauvignon – more dry than sweet wines. What are your customers telling you?

Dennise: The tasting room has been open for ten years and in the early years, the people would say they liked dry wines and then buy sweet. That is changing, especially in the last few years.

Kip: There is still a lot of skepticism amongst wine drinkers and retailers about our ability to grow those grapes that make a good dry red wine. But we've had enough validation from very knowledgeable people in the industry to know we're on the right track. The 2005 Vin du Rio, which is a Bordeaux blend, I priced at $28 and it sold out. So there are some really WOW red wines coming out of Lone Oak Vineyard Estate.

WOW, so not only can grapes be grown from those slopes in Grass Lake but also there's great wines in them there hills - much thanks and L.O.V.E. to you.

PENTAMERE WINERY
The Hole In The Floor Gang

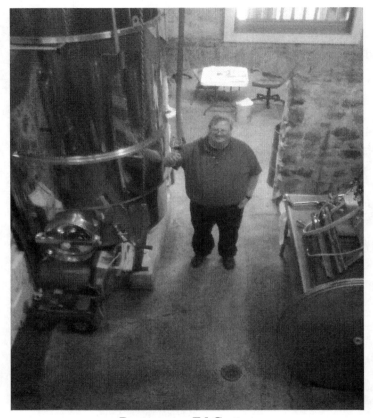

Pentamere - Ed Gerten

The first thing you realize is Pentamere Winery in right in the middle of downtown Tecumseh, Michigan. Upon entering the quaint looking storefront, the second thing you notice as you approach the tasting bar is a BIG hole in the floor. It may be an urban winery but this is truly a fully functioning winery – realized as you gaze at the tanks of wine and bottling machinery below.

Many years ago in the land of Pentamere...ok, it started twelve miles down the road when three guys became best friends as freshmen at Adrian College. Dan Measel (music), Ed Gerten (business) and Nathan Sparks (chemistry) formed a lifelong bond as teenagers and it grows stronger with each great wine they share made from their very own winery. "When someone asks if Pentamere is a family-owned winery, I actually have to pause before answering because my first instinct is to say yes," chuckled Ed.

After graduation, the three amigos all got jobs and took diverse paths out into the world but rarely went a month without contact. The nexus for a winery began when they got together to tackle a new project –making wine. Soon, their bottled wine became Christmas presents and friends began asking about purchasing their creations. "We found ourselves giving away more wine than we were drinking," laughed Ed. "We couldn't sell it so we started teaching others how to make it – until that became overwhelming."

They gravitated to an annual fall 'Crush Party', which eventually stopped their large home winemaking operation when they realized they were hauling 1,800 lbs. of west Michigan grapes and 350 gallons of juice to the party – this was getting well beyond personal consumption! Comments from friends and family spurred Dan and his wife Maria to investigate opening a winery.

After they attended the Midwest Traveling Wine College, a search for the proper venue in southeast Michigan began. They eventually settled on the concept of an urban winery model and picked a downtown commercial property in Tecumseh. It took fourteen months to renovate a former restaurant and open the doors as Pentamere Winery – Michigan's first urban winery in 2002.

The division of labor is far from rigid but equitable – Dan is the winemaker, Ed handles winery operations and retail, Nate is the chemist and Dan's wife Maria does marketing and well, everyone answers to her. The wine selection is diverse and represents the Great Lakes watershed, just as their labels indicate.

Interview with Ed Gerten:

Give us a quick history of this great building.

Ed: It was built in 1872 as a dry grocery store and remained so for the next 50 years. Then it was a clothing store until the late 40's and reopened as Larry's Diner. In 1970 the Chicilean House Spanish Foods Restaurant moved in and on days when the windows fog up you can still read remnants of their sign in the window.

Where did the name Pentamere come from?

Ed: We thought of many names but none of them really clicked. Another college friend suggested Pentamere, which roughly translated means five lakes. We all said 'hey, that sounds pretty good.' Dan came up with our motto 'wines from the vines of the Great Lakes' and we all agreed that was the name for us. We've since discovered the Society for Creative Anachronism calls Michigan 'the Kingdom of Pentamere' and even their maps show this region of southeast Michigan as the Duchy of

Pentamere. Of course, we were immediately paranoid about getting sued but they were actually thrilled (laughing).

What are the advantages and disadvantages of an urban winery?

Ed: The definition of an urban winery is a winery specifically located in a downtown business district for the commercial production of wine. The advantages are we're open the year-round, we're right in the downtown area and we get a lot of foot traffic. The disadvantages – we're open the year-round, are in the downtown area and sometimes we don't get a lot of foot traffic (laughing). It really has worked out well for us though. We've become known as the winery with the hole in the floor.

Which leads me to the next question...there's a big hole in the floor – why?

Ed: It truly was the only way we could get our tanks into the basement. We built a ramp out of the floor joists that were taken out and it took 10 guys to lower the biggest tank. It's a typical Michigan basement with six-foot ceilings, which didn't give us enough room and the stairway down was barely passable for humans. When we're in bottling production we get quite a crowd gathering around 'the hole' to watch.

Is it an Adrian College collaborative effort in naming your wines?

Ed: Dan and I are nautical 'nuts' so to speak and he is an accomplished sailor. With our Great Lakes heritage and theme, we thought it would be fun to name our wines after shipwrecks from the Great Lakes region – there are over 4,000 to pick from! *Wings of Wind* was our first and is a very popular recreational diving site. We've added others like *Monks Haven* Merlot, *Walk-in-Water* and *Monarch of the Glen*. A couple years ago, we made a blush and needed a name, so I started researching. My suggestion cracked Dan up so we went with it – *Betchawanna Blush*.

Describe Dan the winemaker.

Ed: He is an artist. I have the luxury of selling his artwork. Winemaking is art and science together. He describes me as knowing just enough to be dangerous – he's tenacious, too. *Walk-in-Water* started out as a five red wine blend Dan was making for some friends. He tried several bench trials and it just wasn't coming together, so at the end of the day he just threw the leftover wines into a couple glasses. I came down and took a sip from one of the glasses and said 'hey, I think you've got it.' Well, of course he hadn't recorded the percentages – six weeks and 350 trials later, he FINALLY got it again.

Describe the Pentamere gang with a wine.

Ed: Dan is a big red – he has classic ideas on wine but also understands it's 'dry for show, sweet for dough.' Nate is a Chardonnay – very stable, nose to the grindstone. He can sell the heck out of our wines, very personable but doesn't think he knows anything about wine when he really does. Maria is our champagne. She is very classy – knows marketing and is very comfortable in a lot of situations. I'm a Pinot Noir – I like the traditional wines but I also like the young, fruity 'hey, let's do something different' wine.

Where do you see Pentamere winery in the future?

Ed: We've actually outgrown our capacity here so we've acquired a new location for inventory and additional tank space. In the short term, I see us continuing to grow to meet the current demand and gradually increase our presence in the retail market. We're producing between 1,400 to 1,800 cases annually, which is still considered a 'boutique' winery. Ten years down the road, I'd like to think our wine brain trust can come up with enough great wines to get Pentamere over 5,000 cases per year.

Last question – assuming an urban winery draws a diverse crowd…what's the strangest question you've been asked?

Ed: During our first Pioneer Trail wine event, a gentleman came in and asked me my recommendation for a wine pairing with Cheese Whiz. I looked right at him and said 'Thunderbird!' He said 'that's about right' and then we both started laughing. That's the big thing with us at Pentamere – we take our wines seriously but we don't take ourselves seriously. We've always said we'd lock the doors the day it isn't fun anymore.

Here's to keeping the doors open for many, many more years – thanks Ed.

See the Pentamere ad on page 412.

SANDHILL CRANE VINEYARDS
Don't Go To The Birds – Go To The Wine

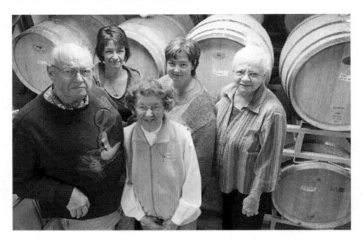

If you're traveling on I-94, between Ann Arbor and Jackson, MI and you love to see birds, take exit 145 and follow the signs to Sandhill Crane Vineyards. Oh sure, there's a bird sanctuary right up the road but you'll wanna try the wine first.

Sandhill Crane Vineyards is aptly named because in the spring and fall you'll see plenty of their namesakes. But the year-round, you can stop in, enjoy some great wine in the tasting room, try a little food from the Crane Café and meet the Moffatt clan.

Norm Moffatt, a retired Detroit policeman, dabbled in making homemade wine for nearly a half century and as he was quoted one day, it became "a hobby run amok." With the purchase of land in the Jackson area and turning cornfields into rows of grapevines, his hobby became an official winery, opening in 2003.

He and his wife Alice made it truly a family owned and operated business by partnering with sister-in-law Anne Leisinger, Heather Price (daughter & business manager) and Holly Balansag (daughter & winemaker). The boutique winery started small but as the people 'flocked' in, the need to enlarge the facility became apparent.

In 2010, they added the café and a banquet room and in 2012, a wraparound porch and major expansion. It has become a destination point for the locals and a regular stop for tourists on the Southeast Michigan Pioneer Wine Trail.

"I never would have dreamed of becoming a winemaker," said Holly. "I moved back from California and offered to help when the idea of building the winery became reality. Seeing the people enjoying my wines in the tasting room gives me great pleasure – I love working at this place my parents created."

And it is a great place to see birds, as well.

Interview with Holly Balansag:

You have been very successful in producing not just popular wines but also award-winning wines, yet you started out with virtually no experience. A leap of faith?

Holly: My father is a great teacher and did a good job tutoring me, but when we started making commercial size batches he turned me loose. I'll admit it was a bit scary at first but I read a lot of books and went to conferences. One of my strong suits is coming from an artistic rather than scientific background, which allows me to think 'outside the box' and get away from traditional blendings. I'd say there was a little luck in there as well (laughing).

There really are a lot of birds around the winery but who came up with the winery name?

Holly: When the property was still farmland and my parents were building their house, we would see a lot of cranes out in the cornfields and there really is a bird sanctuary a couple miles north of here (the Haehnle Memorial Bird Sanctuary). While he was still making homemade wines, my dad would refer to it as his Sandhill Crane winery. We're bird-lovers and the name just felt right.

Of course, you have a picture of cranes on your vineyard logo but who designs your labels?

Holly: I have a degree in photography, so I've taken a few of the pictures. My daughter designed the labels for a couple of the fun wines but my sister Heather does must of the designing. Naming the wines is done by committee – we'll sit around and brainstorm, while enjoying a little wine – but not too much, because the names just keep getting crazier.

You're using cork for your closure. Why?

Holly: Mostly, it's tradition. We use two types – one is completely natural, which is used with the dry reds that are going to be aged. For everything else, we use a composite cork. I've found with the synthetic corks, they're either too hard to get out of the bottle or too easy. Twist-off caps are becoming popular. It eliminates storage problems and cork taint but I'm still in love with the ambiance of a cork and that popping sound when it comes out of the bottle.

How would you characterize your wine list?

Holly: For a small winery we offer a good variety of wines, some years up to 40 different types. I make the traditional ones but as we've grown, I've added more exotic flavored wines to the list. I think that's probably would we're known for – a large quirky wine list...but not because I'm quirky (laughing).

Ok, give me an example of a quirky wine created by Holly.

Holly: One that I hit on early was a wine we call Rhapsody in Red. I blended a red wine with about 20% raspberry wine and made it semi-sweet. Originally, there were a lot of heads shaking around here but it really clicked with people and has turned out to be one of our most popular wines.

What percentage of grapes do you grow at the Vineyards?

Holly: Only about 10% of our grapes are grown here. And that won't change unless we purchase more land. But we do use 100% Michigan fruit. I've stuck with southwest Michigan growers primarily because they have a bit longer growing season and it's easier and less expensive to buy close to home. The overall quality of Michigan fruits is fantastic and always getting better.

When you give a wine tour, what are the most common questions you get?

Holly: Probably, 'how long does the process take?' Many people are confused about fermentation. They don't understand it takes place in about a week and then they ask 'so why do you have to age reds for two years?' Someone always asks how much the oak barrels cost – that's usually followed by shocked looks when I tell them a good French oak barrel costs about $800!

What's the most difficult or frustrating part of your job?

Holly: When I try something new and thought I did everything right and an unexpected problem comes up with the wine, which thankfully doesn't happen very often. Wine is very forgiving. And Michigan winters are a blessing because I can actually stop and take a breath. During the harvest season, I'm going 24/7 and get exhausted but I'll admit, I love what I'm doing and when I see the end results, it rejuvenates me.

A little wine , a little bird watching - works for me. Thanks Holly.

SANDY SHORES WINERY
It Was Meant To Be

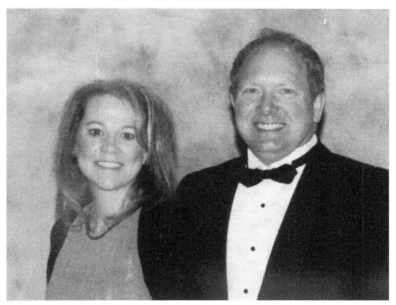

Charlie Ruthruff worked at an orchard not far from his hometown of Charlotte for three years prior to attending Northwood University. Lori picked fruit from the nearby McCallum Orchard growing up in Port Huron and then went off to college at Northwood.

Charlie left as Lori was coming in. After graduation, Lori moved away from Port Huron, as Charlie was moving there. So how did they eventually get married, buy McCallum Orchard and start a winery?

They finally met through mutual friends. "She thought she had escaped Port Huron but I brought her right back," said Charlie. It was meant to be.

After traveling the Midwest, he found a business opportunity when the McCallum Orchard came up for sale. "I had a good working knowledge of the fruit growing industry but I had to learn how to be a farmer (laughing)."

"We finalized the paperwork to buy the orchard one week before we got married. I had to move my stuff back to Port Huron and was starting a new teaching job in the fall. It was a crazy time," admitted Lori.

The McCallum Orchard had been in business for nearly 90 years before the Ruthruffs took charge. Charlie bought everything including the well-established name in 2003. In 2010, they added the Sandy Shores Winery to the operation.

"Charlie is the creative guy and he was thinking about adding the winery within a year. I kept thinking 'we're still learning the orchard business and now he wants to start a winery' (Charlie – 'she's my voice of reason!'). But it's all worked out very well and we've really expanded our customer base," Lori said.

The McCallum Orchard and Cider Mill features a fruit market, a related item store, a you-pick-em orchard, a cider mill and now the Sandy Shores Winery.

Interview with Charlie and Lori Ruthruff:

What or who inspired the winery?

Charlie: Actually, it was Mike Beck at Uncle John's Cider Mill who was instrumental in helping get Sandy Shores Winery off the ground. I was attending an industry meeting and he asked me why I hadn't started up a winery – I had everything he had at Uncle John's. It really made sense. The paperwork just took a few years. I realized, after having a bumper crop of pears one year that you can only sell so many bushels and there was a lot of waste. I was paying workers to pick the fruit and paying them to haul the unsold ones back out to the orchard for fertilizer. The winery solved that problem.

Where did the name Sandy Shores Winery come from?

Charlie: We wanted something simple and easy to spell. With the name Ruthruff, we inherited that problem (laughing). Our home sits right on a sandy shore and my mother's name was Sandy.

Lori: Once we thought it through, Sandy Shores really stuck and all the other potential names were quickly discarded.

How did the logo develop?

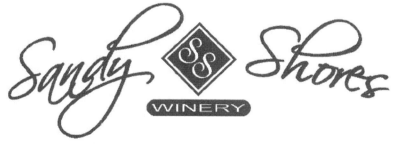

Charlie: We hired a local business to do some sign work and T-shirts for us – so we had them work on a label design. It has a little fancier script writing than the orchard signs. The interesting element we added was a color-coding system with each fruit wine label. Our apple wine has a red label, the pear wine is green, the apricot wine is orange and so forth. We are also bottling almost on demand, which keeps everything fresh and we can spot which wine is selling well at a glance.

Lori: Actually, our customers like the simplicity and straight forwardness of the labeling system. We've had great feedback.

You use that straight forward approach in naming your wines as well.

Charlie: Yes, it is what it is. We grow all ten of the fruits used in our wines right in our orchard. The apple, pear and cherry wines are the stellar ones right now. In the future, when we start blending, we'll come up with some creative names for our new wines.

Why did you decide to go with a smaller 375 ml bottle?

Charlie: Again, it was Mike Beck who told us the most important part of marketing your product is to get the customer to try it. We felt people would take home a variety of smaller bottled wines instead of just one or two 750 ml bottles.

Lori: In many cases, a person will sample a wine they've never tried before – really like it – then buy one for themselves and one for a friend to try.

You went with screw caps for the smaller bottles. Why?

Charlie: As it turned out, our bottle source only came with that option. We were also told because of the sugar content in fruit wines, a traditional cork invariably gets 'welded' into the bottle and breaks off when extracted. When our customers started requesting the 750 ml bottles, which we started using in 2012, we went to a bar top or 'scork', which seals well and you don't need a corkscrew.

What is the most common question you get in the tasting room and the most unique?

Charlie: Many of our customers are really into 'buy Michigan' and they will ask 'do you make the wine here?' and 'do you grow the fruit here?' and 'are you the winemaker?' and I get to answer with a smile 'yes, yes and yes.' The most 'unique' question was when a lady asked me 'what grapes do you use to make your cherry wine?' That was a real head scratcher (laughing)!

Lori, describe your husband using wine adjectives and Charlie, you describe Lori.

Lori: A good Michigan wine is as sweet and flavorful my husband has been since we've been together.

Charlie: The word spicy immediately comes to mind because she's a fighter and digs in to help with whatever needs to get done and still has a full-time job. So, I would say spicy, smooth and crisp – all together, it makes a unique wine and she is a unique person.

When you put the two together, it's a combination that's hard to beat – the Ruthruffs and Sandy Shores Winery – thanks to you both.

See the Sandy Shores ad on page 415.

UNCLE JOHN'S FRUIT HOUSE WINERY
With Uncle Mike Beck At The Helm

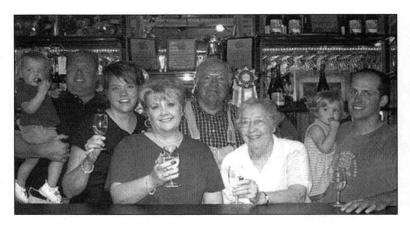

There has been a Beck fruit farm in St. Johns, Michigan since great-great grandfather Frank Beck started growing apples there in late 1880's. Of course, he probably never envisioned the big white barn becoming an iconic sight and tourist destination along U.S. 27 either. It's much more than a farm and cider mill. Since 2003, guests have been able to stop into the Fruit House Winery for a sample of Beck's world-class hard cider.

Not only did the farm become a major apple supplier but they also were one of the largest suppliers of beeswax to the U.S. Army during WWII – at the time, one of the main sources of waterproofing. By the late 1960's, John Beck had taken charge of the orchard operation but it was rapidly becoming difficult to turn a profit in the wholesale apple business. The Becks needed to diversify.

Thanks to the advice from an MSU Cooperative Extension Agent, they began to concentrate on the 'value added' retail side.

"Our commodity was apples for wholesale but we changed the focus and expanded the use of apples," said fifth generation farmer Mike Beck. "We started making cider, pies, caramel apples, wine, etc."

Today, it's not unusual to see a line of cars, buses and travel vans turning into Uncle John's. "It seems every year, our orchard gets smaller and the parking area gets bigger," said Mike.

Interview with Mike Beck:

Uncle John is actually your father, the fourth generation Beck to run the Beck orchard. But how did the farm get the name Uncle John's Cider Mill?

Mike: There wasn't any in-depth marketing research done, I can tell ya (laughing). A bunch of his nieces and nephews were helping him clean out the big barn to convert it into a cider mill. They said 'what are you gonna call the cider mill Uncle John?' It kinda rolled off their tongues and stuck – very scientific don't ya think?

It has grown into a destination point with a multitude of activities. Tell us about that progression.

Mike: I can show you old pictures of the roadside stands but Uncle John's truly is an entertainment center for the family – plenty of things for the kids to do while mom & dad sample the cider or shop. Believe it or not, we may have been one of the very first in the entire country to do a corn maze back in the late 1980's – we were inspired by the hedge maze in the movie The Shining. Now, they are everywhere. No apple goes to waste either. The best ones go into our hard ciders but even the unworthy apples get used – we built a big slingshot so people could shoot 'em at targets.

What is the process you use to come up with the names of your hard ciders?

Mike: We are the 'simpletons' of naming products – it's pretty straightforward – the name is what you're getting. For example, we make a premium hard cider using exclusively Russet apples and call it... Russet. Another premium hard cider made with American and English apples, we named Melded, which is about as fancy as I get. I refuse to make a product that I can't pronounce (laughing).

Is there a preference in the type of closure you're using?

Mike: We use a synthetic cork and I've never had a problem. But if I had the equipment, I'd go to twist caps in a heartbeat. All of the premium wines in New Zealand and quite a few in California are going in that direction.

I'm assuming each variety of apple gives the wine or cider a distinct flavor but how many varieties of apple are there?

Mike: I use primarily a dozen different varieties for my ciders and, yes, each has a very different flavor. But I've got probably 50 different varieties right here on the farm. In the United States there are probably 3,000 and worldwide, maybe double that number. And those are just the named ones. One bee pollinates different trees, several bees pollinate the same tree – all the apples are just a little bit different – that's the wonder of cross pollinated fruit and brings out the wonderful flavors in our ciders.

So, there is cider, hard cider and apple wine. What is the difference?

Mike: Around the world, cider would be alcoholic but in North America cider is the term used for fresh juice. When talking with other winemakers, we use the term cider and imply that it has alcohol. Americans generally have accepted the term hard cider to have alcohol in it (6-9%). Adding sugar adds to the alcohol content to make apple wine (10-14%).

Although hard cider has been around for centuries, it seems like a recent discovery in the wine industry, especially here in Michigan. Is this true?

Mike: It IS the biggest trend in the alcohol beverage industry – that may sound a bit prejudiced – well, sure I am. But the fact is hard cider has shown over 20% growth each of the last four years and a 50% rise in the last six months of 2012.

To what do you attribute to this dramatic upturn?

Mike: Michigan is actually poised to be the great cider hotbed. We bring more varieties up to commercial production than any other state. There are larger apple growing regions. Washington is the largest by far but they concentrate on the 'pretty apples' for the grocery store – the Red Delicious, Golden Delicious, Granny Smith and Galas. New York produces more but primarily in McIntosh varieties – Cortland, Spartan & Empire. We have at least 40 commercial varieties – Michigan has so much more diversity to use in cider production. That's why our ciders are the best.

So, use a nice wine to describe yourself.

Mike: I'm a Cabernet Sauvignon – big, bold...I was going to say understated but I've never had a Cabernet that was understated and no one would believe I was either (laughing).

I'll toast a big, bold hard cider to you. Thanks Mike.

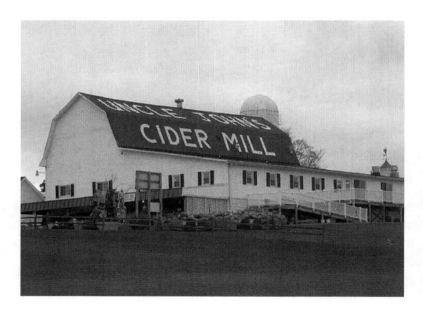

See Uncle John's Fruit House Winery Ad on page 417.

YOOPER WINE

MACKINAW TRAIL..325
NORTHERN SUN WINERY................................331

MACKINAW TRAIL WINERY
Just when I thought I was out, the wine pulled me back in.

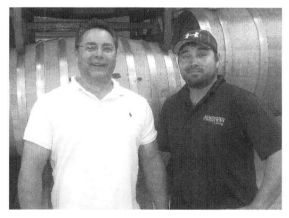

Raffaele and Dustin Stabile

Raffaele (Ralph) Stabile was born and raised on the east side of Detroit. His grandfather had a small vineyard and each fall the family would gather for the harvest and make the wine. He was the one to carry on the family tradition but he never thought it would go this far – a trail of wineries and tasting rooms all across northern Michigan.

As a young teenager, Ralph moved to the Upper Peninsula when his father bought a small resort in 1979. "It was a culture shock and I hated the U.P.," he said. "Someone once asked me how I got over moving up there and I told him I'm still not over it (laughing)."

One good thing about the move up north was meeting his future wife Laurie (married over thirty years now). They got married in 1983, tried college for a year, and then Ralph joined the military for a four-year stint. After eventually settling in Chicago, he began a career in the telecommunications industry.

In 1993, the company opened a position in the U.P. "This time I went back willingly," Ralph said. "It was closer to the family and I started making wine again." Early in the new millennium, after the 'bubble burst,' he saw the handwriting on the wall and in 2003 made the decision to become a full-time winemaker. "My wife says I'm anal, I say I'm analytical," Ralph chuckled. "I just started reading and researching everything about winemaking that I could get my hands on."

Soon after incorporating in 2004, they bought the old fishery on the Manistique River and opened the Mackinaw Trail Winery tasting room in 2005. A second tasting room was opened in Mackinaw City in 2007 when 'I realized the romantic notion of sitting around a wine barrel sipping on our product doesn't pay the bills.'

With another leap of faith, the Stabiles opened yet another tasting room in downtown Petoskey in 2009. It soon became apparent there was a need for more room so Ralph and his son Dustin started looking at land below the bridge to expand. They searched for the right property in the Traverse area – on both peninsulas - and in southwest Michigan.

On a trip back home, they took US 131 north out of Cadillac. "As we got just south of Petoskey, I spotted an empty field," Ralph recalled. "I climbed the hill, looked down and envisioned our new winery. Of course, the property wasn't for sale. Remember the old adage – everything is for sale – well, I'm not saying 'I made 'em an offer they couldn't refuse' but I am Italian (laughing)."

"Actually, the timing was right and I gave them a fair offer. We closed on the property in February 2012, broke ground in June 2012 and had our grand opening for the new winery in June 2013." Timing is everything and it doesn't hurt to be a full-speed-ahead Italian, either.

Interview with Ralph Stabile:

Were you the pioneer of winemaking in the U.P.?

Ralph: I wouldn't say we were the pioneers. There is a large population of Italians in the Iron Mountain area who have been making wine probably since 1900. I remember the year I moved up here, there were 150 cars parked at the railroad station to pick up their shipments of grapes from California to go back home and make the wine. But I was the first licensed winery in the U.P.

So what is it with Italians and wine – if you cut their veins, does Chianti come out?

Ralph: It's part of our heritage. I grew up watching my grandfather get the grapes and make the wine when I was very young, then I was right in there helping when I got older. For me, it still goes back to the old country. I've got relatives in Sicily who own vineyards and a winery. It's funny looking back now, because I really have been doing this my whole life. Of course, I went through my young adult 'trial and error' period but one day it just dawned on me 'hey, why am I looking for a job – this is what I was born to do.'

How did you come up with the name Mackinaw Trail?

Ralph: I wanted to grab something unique and recognizable by region. Ironically, the road the winery is on outside of Petoskey is called Mackinaw Trail.

You were technical in your other career – does that help you as a winemaker?

Ralph: It helps from an analytical standpoint. That's my mindset. I was the kid that was tearing things apart to see how they worked but unfortunately, I never took the time to put things back together. My personality fits this business – digging deep to learn and understand. Every year is different. You may be making the same wines but each vintage is unique.

One of your Rieslings is made 'in a Germanic fashion.' What does that mean?

Ralph: There are several ways to make a sweetened Riesling. The Germanic way is to stop the fermentation prior to the wine going completely dry, which leaves residual sugars in the wine. Another way is to ferment to dryness and add Riesling juice back in to sweeten it up. You can also ferment to dryness and sweeten it up with plain sugar. I've tried it all three ways before.

Who shot the deer that's on your label of Big Red?

Ralph: (laughing) That actually is a stag shot by a friend of mine – I think it was out in Maine. It's our house red and everyone likes it.

Explain how you choose barrels for aging your reds.

Ralph: First, you custom order barrels from a cooper. To me, it's all about layers – each layer provides some component that makes up the wine. American oak gives you caramelly, vanilla tones. But it can be overpowering, so we use a smaller percentage of American. Fifty percent of our barrels are French oak, which gives the wine spicey tones. Hungarian oak is basically a happy medium. You add it all together to produce a unique quality product.

Give us the history of your original winery in Manistique and the tasting rooms in Mackinaw City and Petoskey.

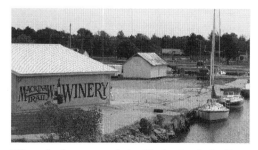

Ralph: The Manistique building had been a fishery for over 100 years, right on the Manistique River, which flows out to Lake Michigan. The whole area originally looked similar to old Fishtown (Leland) on Leelanau peninsula. Our tasting room is in an old net storage building out at the end of the pier – we call it the Tin Shed Tasting Room. In Mackinaw City, there's an outdoor mall called Mackinaw Crossings that was built back in the 1990's – we leased some space there. It has an Italian motif. Our tasting room in downtown Petoskey is in the gaslight district – it's a vibrant old downtown.

Are you going to stay open the year-round with any of your locations?

Ralph: The Petoskey area gets a lot of skiers in the winter so we'll keep the winery and downtown tasting room open. The Mackinaw City location does great and is open from May to October. The Manistique operation will stay open until the New Year and then close for three months.

And now you've got a new home base in Petoskey and are a part of the new Bay View Wine Trail.

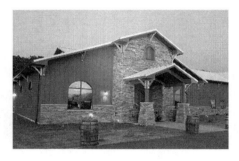

Ralph: The new winery is 8,500 sq. ft. and will position us to grow for quite a few years. There are a bunch of new wineries in the Petoskey/Harbor Springs area, which has tremendous growth potential. We are all working together to improve everyone's wine quality. I'm glad to help where I can and hopefully stop the new ones from making the same mistakes I did (laughing).

We're glad the Italian in you wouldn't let you get out – thanks Ralph.

See the Mackinaw Trail ad on page 410.

NORTHERN SUN WINERY
It Takes a Long Day To Make Good Wine

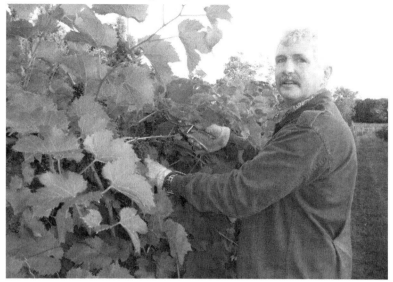

When people hear about living north of the bridge, the Mackinaw Bridge, they expect to here about cold days and long winter nights. They don't expect to hear about eighteen hours of sunlight and grapes that make wonderful wines. Don't believe it? Then you need to visit Northern Sun Winery just west of Escanaba.

Dave Anthony is a born and bred Yooper from Marquette in the Upper Peninsula. He went to college at Northern Michigan University. Straight out of school, he went to work for U.S. Senator Carl Levin. Twelve years later, he took his own path to public policy in 1990 by getting elected to the Michigan House of Representatives.

While serving in Lansing, Dave co-chaired the Committee on Agriculture with a grape farmer. It also happens, there is a large constituency of Italians in his district. This led to many invitations to tour home wine cellars and basement winemaking operations.

Consequently, Dave put in an order for California grapes and made wine in the basement of his fiancés Lansing home. "For a long time we played with making wine," Dave said. "We had some successes but a lot of failures too (laughing)." That didn't deter them from getting married in 1999 and that same year he took his bride Susie back north to work for one of the tribal communities near Escanaba.

The idea of living in the country appealed to the Anthonys, so they bought a farm in Bark River. "We had no intentions of starting a winery but I did want to try growing grapes, " Dave recalled. "My first vines came from a winemaker's grape packet and understandably didn't do well."

"I started consulting with MSU but unfortunately they all thought I lived in the sub-artic and just knew grapes couldn't grow there. Eventually, they steered me to French hybrid varieties, which are considered cool climate grapes. After more research, I discovered the University of Minnesota viticultural program, as well as the Marquette and LaCresent grapes."

Soon, he was also planting more varieties and the idea of starting a winery began to take hold. That plan was accelerated once the vines matured and they had more grapes - a lot of grapes. In 2009, Dave started investing in equipment for a winemaking operation and the Northern Sun Winery opened in 2011.

About ten miles west of Escanaba off US-41/US-2, you'll find a quaint little tasting room. Susie and Smity will probably greet you. You'll probably also see Dave's 86-year-old father, Robert, out tending to the vineyards. Like his son, he has a passion for wine because he rarely misses a day.

Interview with Dave Anthony:

So your winery is in the land of the northern sun – resulting in the name of the winery?

Dave: We actually believe there is an advantage to living this far north. With the extended daylight, we can work until nearly 11:00 pm for many days in June. The vines take advantage of that extra sunlight and grow like crazy – hence, the name Northern Sun Winery.

Who designed the tasting room?

Dave: I designed it from an old 1917 European photograph of a country villa. I made the rooflines similar to what you would see in the Mediterranean culture. It's only about 400 sq. ft. but people seem to like the cozy atmosphere.

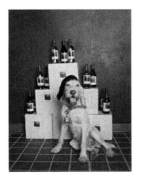

Tell us about your 'fanciful' wine dog.

Dave: Smity is the Princess of Northern Sun. She follows Susie everywhere and of course, gets the Princess treatment and is spoiled terribly. Her name comes from the movie *Roman Holiday* with Audrey

Hepburn and Gregory Peck. It's about a royal Princess who hides her true identity with the nickname 'Smity.' The dog is actually a Spinore Italiano, which is an Italian bird dog, but she's our Princess in disguise.

You served on the Michigan Grape and Wine Industry Council from 2006 to 2010. What was the best thing you learned?

Dave: Without a doubt, it offered me an opportunity to have discussions with farmers and winemakers who introduced me to concepts that were based on practical, hands on experience – things from a business point of view instead of being academically oriented - things you would never hear at a conference.

How big a difference is there between the climate in Bark River and the Traverse wine region?

Dave: Surprisingly, there isn't a big difference because our property is located in a micro-climate, which insulates us a little bit from the harsh winters in the U.P. I keep a close eye on the heat units, which is a measurement of growing degree days. We're step in step with Leelanau and Old Mission peninsulas right up to mid-September. That's when I start having minor frost incidents. The Traverse area avoids those with their lake effect. My hybrid grapes are fully ripened by the first of October and their French vinifera will need a few more weeks.

Were you aware of the micro-climate before you purchased your farm?

Dave: It was dumb luck (laughing). Not only that, but after making the decision to try growing grapes, the research said land with a gradual incline is more suitable and sandy loam soil is preferred – I have both. It was dumb luck but I'll take it.

Where does your customer base come from?

Dave: The majority are local or from the central U.P. I would estimate about 45% are tourists. But our guest book has names from New Zealand and quite a few from California, so they're finding us.

Have you acquired a winemaking philosophy?

Dave: We don't bottle anything unless we grow it. To me, that's the traditional approach to viticulture. When you grow your own fruit, it gives you more control and allows you to work with the very best fruit you have.

What has been the most satisfying part of owning a winery?

Dave: The most surprising and satisfying aspect from a grower/winemaker standpoint has been winning competitions. When you get people who are standouts in the wine industry proclaiming your product to be award winning, that's enough to make my week. We've won in California, New York, Indiana and even right here in Michigan. I've been told when our wines were revealed, it's raised a few eyebrows and caused a commotion. That just makes my smile bigger.

They've just never experienced that northern sun and a good Upper Peninsula wine before – thanks, Dave.

VINE TO DINE

HAVE WINE – WILL WRITE 337
　Authors of the From The Vine and History of Michigan Wines – Lorri Hathaway & Sharon Kegerreis

THERE'S TIERS IN YOUR WINE 343
　Sommelier Tom Fischer

STARTING A VINEYARD 347
　Dave Zimmerman

DISTRIBUTORS 351
　Fabiano Brothers – Gordy Dalziel

RETAILERS 357
　Brew Krew 357
　Dusty's Cellar 361
　Eastman Party Store 366
　Ideal Party Store 371

HAVE WINE – WILL WRITE

Authors of the *From The Vine* and *The History of Michigan Wines* books, Lorri Hathaway & Sharon Kegerreis

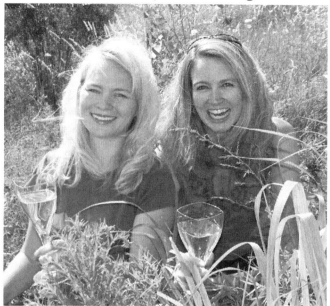

They both grew up in northern Michigan and both graduated from Central Michigan University but never crossed paths until they met while working in Lansing many years later.

Lorri is a native of the Leelanau peninsula but grew up while the wine industry there was very small. After obtaining a college degree in business, she spent much of her time in commercial real estate. Sharon is from Charlevoix and her CMU communications degree took her to Colorado, then California and eventually back to Michigan. In the corporate world, they met through a business leads group and hit it off immediately.

Ironically, they met their future husbands through the same group.

Both had a passion for writing and a secret desire to write a book. After chucking the corporate life, they re-discovered Michigan wines and started a company together, called Michigan Vine, which promoted the industry and involved putting on wine events.

What started out as a collaboration to write a 'simple wine guide' evolved in a contract to write the coffee table sized book *From The Vine*, which was published in 2007. Along the way, they began writing articles for the Michigan Grape and Wine Industry Council and the *Michigan Wine Country* magazine. That led to writing another book in 2010 called *The History of Michigan Wines*.

While researching *From The Vine*, Lorri and Sharon personally talked with all 51 wineries in the state. In recent years, that number has exploded and currently there are over 100 wineries in Michigan.

Lorri is back living in Traverse City to freelance write and work as Director of Marketing, Communications and Media Relations for the Leelanau Peninsula Wine Trail. Sharon is freelance writing and working on books. Although they have moved on to other projects, their commitment to Michigan wines remains unwavering. Their knowledge and insights into the Michigan wine industry are priceless. Oh, what stories they can tell.

Interview with Lorri Hathaway and Sharon Kegerreis:

Where did your love of wine come from?

Lorri: I was a beer drinker in college, but in my mid-20s, I was working as a commercial real estate broker and joined a wine club. Then, I began exploring Michigan wines and my palate evolved to where I now enjoy a wide range of varietals.

Sharon: While in California, I did a lot of 'wine & dine' with my job and traveled internationally in areas where wine was served at practically every meal. After returning to Michigan, I discovered Michigan winemakers were crafting some really great wines.

You came up with this idea for a book – how did you find a publisher?

Lorri: Our simple wine guide was turning into multiple pages for each winery. We became fascinated with each winemaker's story. We got very lucky and it's not the typical way it's supposed to happen, especially for first time authors. Sharon made one phone call.

Sharon: I almost feel guilty because we have no story about our struggle to find a publisher. I called Ann Arbor Media Group and pitched our idea. They loved it, said yes, and then said you've got six months!

What was the division of labor in writing the book?

Lorri: Every story went back and forth until we were both satisfied, so it was a true collaboration. I'm the facts person – she's the creative person looking for the right story angle. It was a frantic six months and by the time we finished, I don't think we talked to each other for a month (laughing).

Sharon: The photography was probably 50-50 as well. We took over 5,000 pictures – thank goodness for the delete button on our digital cameras (laughing). The cool thing is we each have our strengths in writing and worked those ideas into the project. I think we brought out the best in each other.

What was the most interesting thing you learned along the way?

Lorri: One thing that fascinated me was 'ice wine' and how it is made. It's an intense harvest, a lot of hard work and such a huge risk for the wineries, and that's one of the reasons why it's pricey. Overall, Michigan winemakers are very hardworking farmers.

Sharon: I found the "perceived versus reality" image of the winemaker to be enlightening. They truly are stewards of the land. They love getting their hands dirty, battling Mother Nature and crafting high-quality wine. Their friendly demeanor was a real pleasant surprise.

Who was the most surprising or interesting person you met?

Lorri: The first person that comes to mind is Ed O'Keefe at Chateau Grand Traverse. He's had a fascinating life and had a huge impact on northern Michigan's wine industry.

Sharon: If I ever need a great quote for an article, I call Bryan Ulbrich or Larry Mawby. They are both incredibly knowledgeable, make excellent wine and are so poetic in the way they talk about wine. I'm also in awe of pioneer winemakers Bernie Rink and Doug Welsch.

There are many beautiful vineyards in Michigan but what was the most breathtaking view?

Lorri: Well, I got married at Ciccone Vineyards on Leelanau peninsula so I'm a bit partial to that view – it's beautiful. On Old Mission, I enjoy Chateau Chantal where you can see the bay in two directions.

Sharon: I agree with Chateau Chantal and I also admire the views offered by 2 Lads and Brys Estate.

Switching to your *History of Michigan Wines* book, in your opinion, what was one of the most significant events in our wine history?

Lorri: I think looking back at the days of Prohibition, the wine industry never stopped due to extensive bootlegging across the Detroit River. When Prohibition ended, the wine industry exploded because established wineries relocated from Windsor to Detroit and the flourishing vineyards from the prominent grape juice industry here.

Sharon: In the early, early years, wine tended to be fortified – it was made sweet to appeal to consumers post-war and post Great Depression. Eventually, Michigan produced table wines, beginning with a Baco Noir by Bronte. However, Ed O'Keefe boldly planted only European Vinifera grape varietals on Old Mission Peninsula, disproving that "only French-American hybrid wines" could grow in Michigan's cold climate. Chateau Grand Traverse remains a cornerstone in the industry today.

What was the most interesting fact you learned about our wine industry?

Lorri: I was totally surprised to learn Michigan was ranked 3rd in the nation in wine production for the three decades after Prohibition. It didn't just surprise us, it has surprised a lot of people in the industry. Unfortunately, state regulations and fees challenged the industry and a slow reaction to a changing preference of the American wine drinker hurt the state's wine industry.

Sharon: I found it interesting that southeast Michigan was the commercial hub of the industry back in the late 1800s. And long before this, explorers like LaSalle and Cadillac crafted wine using the bounty of wild grapes in the area.

Did writing these books change your wine palate?

Lorri: One thing I learned while tasting at Michigan wineries is to be open-minded – don't dismiss table wines or wines with funky names just because they aren't named by a European vinifera or French-American hybrid varietal. You'll find some great wines with crazy names out there.

Sharon: I was never really into sweet wines. I've grown to love dry Michigan Rosés for summertime. I'm probably a seasonal wine drinker now. There's a great Michigan wine for every season – so you know I love at least four wine varietals, right (laughing)?

A toast to every season – early spring, spring, late spring, early summer, summer…thanks to you both.

THERE'S TIERS IN YOUR WINE
MICHIGAN'S THREE-TIER DISTRIBUTION SYSTEM

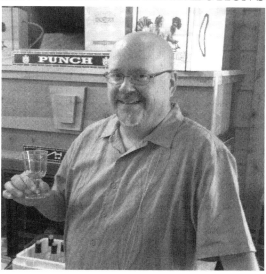

A Brief Overview by Tom Fischer, Sommelier with thirteen years of experience in the wine industry.

From 1918 to 1933, Prohibition brought the non-alcohol beverage era to Michigan. It also brought in the unique distribution system called bootlegging.

Immediately following the repeal of the 18th Amendment, which prohibited the distribution of alcohol, the Michigan Liquor Control Commission started handling the duties of distribution through state-controlled retail stores and began implementing a 3-tier system (producers – distributors – retailers).

Whether the system is fair to consumers is debatable but as Michigan's wine industry has grown, so have the laws and ordinances of the state. The "Three Tier" system has long been a part of these rules and guidelines.

No alcoholic beverage (wine, beer or liquor) produced outside of the state of Michigan may directly sold to any customer inside the state of Michigan. Any product from another state or country must be "imported" into the state through a broker (or manufacturer) to a licensed "Distributor."
.
These distributors in turn will sell the products to licensed retail and restaurant clients, who then sell the products to the end consumer (you and me). Michigan wineries had been held to the same agreement within the state until quite recently.

So, as you can see, there is plenty of room for prices to increase before any alcohol is consumed. The producer sells the product to a distributor, in most cases, for a profit. The distributor adds his profit to the price then sells the product to a retailer or restaurateur. The retailer or restaurateur apply their margins to the product and finally sells the product to the consumer.

Although there is a need for regulation, the system, by its nature, makes for a slow moving and slow reacting bureaucracy. Many times the anticipated release of a new product stalls out and ultimately fails because it gets mired in legal proceedings, and distributor disagreements about territories are common.

Once a winery, brewery, or distillery has signed a contract with a distributor, it is difficult to get out of that agreement, regardless how well or how poorly the distributor performs with the brand. There is a term used in the industry referring to certain distributors as 'contract killers', a term meant to imply a distributor might take on a brand with the intent of making it fail simply through a lack of effort in promoting or limited distribution to prevent competition against a "more important" product the distributor already offers.

Recent legislation now allows Michigan wineries to bypass at least the distribution step of the process. In a 2010 interview with Michigan By The Bottle, Doug Welsch, owner of the Fenn Valley Vineyards addressed the issue of wineries selling directly to consumers and a potential problem on the horizon.

Welsch said, "Right now, we have a wide-open marketing opportunity. We can taste in our tasting rooms, and we can sell and ship directly to the retail consumer. We can sell directly to a restaurant or store without going through a distributor. Or we can sell through a distributor.

"The loss of our ability to self-distribute from the winery to a store/restaurant would put a number of small wineries out of business. Back when direct shipping was an issue (Granholm vs Heald), the distributors, who lobbied HARD against our right to ship wine directly to our customers, inserted a poison pill into the state wine legislation.

"It specifically states that should an outstate producer (winery) want to enjoy the same rights as a Michigan winery, namely to sell directly to a store/restaurant without going through a distributor, and should this end up in court with a ruling that grants an outstate producer the right to self distribute across state lines to a store/restaurant in MI, the poison pill kicks in.

"Then we would immediately loose the right to self distribute. This would stifle the small Michigan winery who has no distributor and would limit them to retail sales only. Even for us larger wineries, that would cause severe pain as we self distribute to a lot of local stores/restaurants that our distributor does not service."

Many Michigan wineries still use distributors to sell their products, because the distributor takes care of all of the transportation, shipping, and logistics of getting the product to market. However, many of the newer and smaller wineries are taking the 'do it yourself' approach.

You had me at 'hello' and lost me when you said 'I don't drink wine.'

STARTING A VINEYARD

DAVE ZIMMERMAN
GOOD WINE STARTS WITH GOOD GRAPES

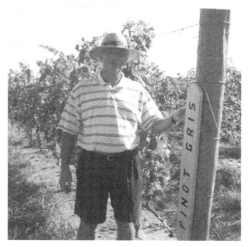

The origins of great wine start with a passion to make a vine grow from the land, which produces a quality grape.

Who is this person who provides the raw materials to make the magic happen? Many times you never see their name on a wine trail or read it on a label or even hear it in conversation.

In this case, it's a retired Detroiter who was told repeatedly his land was perfect for growing grapes. David Zimmerman bought land between Leland and Northport to build a home on and retire, which he did in 2002.

Another Leelanau peninsula winery owner told him his property was a premium site for a vineyard. David ignored him. Then after a neighbor almost insisted he try growing grapes, David admitted 'I kinda backed into this reluctantly and now I'm hooked.'

"I don't have a stellar wine background - my introduction was with drinking Mateus as a teenager and of course, the trendy thing to do was stick a candle in the empty bottle. I graduated from that to Blue Nun but my palate has gotten a little more sophisticated (laughing)."

With his third crop coming in 2013, his talent for growing high-quality grapes gets more sophisticated each year. He sells his grapes to his neighbor at Gills Pier Winery and their winemaker Bryan Ulbrich at Left Foot Charley Winery in Traverse City.

Interview with David Zimmerman:

What grapes have you planted, why and what is the origin?

David: I have 2 acres of Riesling and 1 acre of Pinot Gris. I chose those primarily because Riesling is a world class grape grown here and they both are a cold hardy vine that does well in our climate.

Why did you choose Gills Pier to contract with?

David: There are several reasons - we have a good relationship - they are neighbors and we have a handshake deal. Also, Bryan is the winemaker and he makes a great Riesling and uses my Pinot Gris grapes for a wonderful blend. Although my name wasn't going to be on the bottle, I wanted to say to my friends 'my grapes are in this bottle of wine.' I wouldn't hesitate to put one of those bottles in front of my most discriminating wine drinking friends.

What was the process from the time you decided to try growing grapes to the actual planting?

David: The land was used at one time as pasture and had remained fallow for about 30 years. I cleared and tilled the land with my little tractor. Then I hired a wine consulting company who put in a crop of sorghum and planted rye for a winter cover crop. Both were turned under for green fertilizer before the vines were planted.

Obviously you would be considered a small time grower but is it profitable?

David: From a business standpoint, I'd probably have a more profitable chance at the Casino (laughing). In the long run, I'll cover my expenses and make some money but I do this more for personal satisfaction. Aesthetically it's great to look at and adds a little *panache* to the property.

Is there a big difference in growing Riesling or Pinot Gris?

David: It's interesting that Riesling is a German wine and those wines are very orderly and very structured. The Pinot Gris, being a French varietal, is total chaos and much harder to control. I am not trying to cast aspersions on anyone's ancestry (laughing) - that's just the way it is with growing these grapes.

Who determines the time to pick the grapes?

David: I'll do a sugar content assessment when the grapes are getting close to being ripe. I'll e-mail the information to Bryan and the owner at Gills Pier to let them know. Bryan is looking for the right sugar and mineral levels for his winemaking, which is part science and part art. He looks at his schedule and makes the call when to pick.

Do the grapes go right from the vineyard to the winery?

David: Yes, they are loaded on trucks and immediately shipped down to the Left Foot Charley Winery. It's like watching your babies leave home. The first year, my wife and I followed the trucks down to Traverse City and Bryan gave us a glass of wine as we watched our grapes go into the de-stemmer and then the crusher. There is a sense of relief but it's also an exciting time.

Describe yourself in wine.

David: I enjoy wine, particularly with food, so I would classify myself as a 'drinker' (laughing). Seriously, one of the things I like about our Michigan wines are most of them are right around 10 to 12% alcohol - I enjoy a vodka drink occasionally but not in my wine. So many California wines are bragging about 16% alcohol in their wines and I think it just detracts from the taste. I am a Pinot Noir guy. I hope that doesn't mean it's chaos being around me (laughing).

With a glass of Gills Pier Riesling in hand, you're calm, cool and connected. Thanks David.

DISTRIBUTORS

FABIANO BROTHERS DISTRIBUTOR
This Wines For You

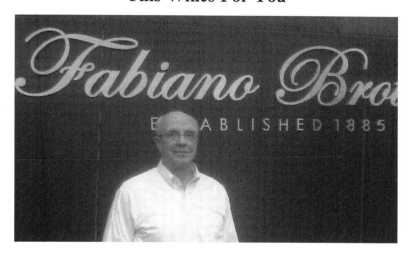

When the Fabiano family opened a business in Italy in 1885, they sold fruit, vegetables and homemade wine. Over 125 years later, they have grown to become the largest Anheuser-Busch distributor under one roof in Michigan. That roof is a new state of the art, 200,000 sq. ft. headquarters facility in Bay City, which opened in 2010. They ditched the produce but still sell wine – lots of wine.

"This is still a family-owned business that has made a huge commitment to the wine industry in Michigan," said Gordy Dalziel, Director of Sales and Marketing - Wine Division at Fabiano's. "We have over 200 North American labels of wine in our portfolio and we're always looking to expand, especially right here in our state. There are exciting new wines being produced all the time in Michigan."

Gordy came to Fabiano Bros. just as they were moving their distribution operation to its new location from Mt. Pleasant where they had opened for business in 1919. He brought over 30 years experience working in the wholesale beverage industry, 23 of them at the E J Gallo Wine Company as a rep for the Upper Peninsula and most of northern Michigan.

"The Gallo and Fabiano companies have similar cultures, strong values and a willingness to give back to the community," said Gordy. "The transition to Fabiano's was smooth – right place and the right time for me."

While working in the Traverse City/Petoskey/Alpena areas, he had an opportunity to observe the wine industry throughout its growing pains and struggle for recognition. "Michigan wineries are dedicated to producing quality wines," he said. "They are starting to get regional support and I see it only getting better."

Gordy's staff is marketing seven different price catalogs in 26 Michigan counties. They are part of a workforce that helped Fabiano Brothers recently receive an Ambassador of Excellence Award in the beverage industry. Through performance, service and Gordy's leadership, Fabiano's continues to put Michigan wines on the wine map of the world.

Interview with Gordy Dalziel:

What do you use for criteria in selecting a wine for your portfolio?

Gordy: First and foremost, we evaluate how stable the company is and obviously, the taste profile. We're also very interested how the wine is packaged and how it fits in our portfolio. We look at how it may affect our current suppliers and what the long-term plans are...where they plan to be in the future.

How has the distribution marketing changed over the years?

Gordy: Wines used to be slow developing but now with the social media, marketing strategies are changing rapidly. You'll see people taking pictures of wines in stores and blogging immediately about pricing – 'I spotted this wine at this retailer for this price' or maybe at a restaurant, 'I'm here at the bar – I tried this wine – good deal, tastes great.' It's amazing how quickly the word spreads.

Are the distributors regulated as intensely as wineries?

Gordy: Yes, in certain areas, such as guidelines in pricing and promotions on or off premise. We have people here who keep everyone in line and our wholesale association keeps us up on the latest that's going on at the state and federal level. We also have our own checks and balances system in place with computerized ordering. For instance, we are restricted as to where we can sell certain wines in particular areas, so if the item is punched in for a non-sale county the computer tells us immediately.

How do you keep all those orders straight?

Gordy: Each wine is coded and the cart takes an employee to the right place in the warehouse to pick up the right number of bottles. It helps reduce what we call 'mispicks.' We're running at about 98% efficiency on correct orders.

What are you seeing that is new and innovative with wines these days?

Gordy: I had someone bring in 'wine in a can' the other day. I haven't tried it yet (laughing) but I'm also not discounting it...yet. Wine by the keg is just becoming a more popular way to sell wine. Places like hotels, restaurants and wine bars are looking into this dispensing method. Good Harbor winery is supplying us with wine in a big cardboard box and it's all eco-friendly without a deposit.

What are you hearing from other distributors about Michigan wines?

Gordy: On the national front, I'm hearing about them becoming a more significant player. Currently, Michigan wines are doing well regionally and many distributors are talking about them being a tremendous opportunity, especially with the recent growth. They are being featured in restaurants in New York and Chicago and we expect them to continue expanding.

What are retailers saying about Michigan wines?

Gordy: Based on the recent growth over the past decade, more and more retailers are jumping on board. Many restaurants and wine bars are starting to feature Michigan wines on a particular night. They understand the importance of promoting locally and in-state produced wines. Retailers are allotting more shelf space to Michigan wines. It's not just the big chain stores either. The independents are doing the same. They're being very supportive and it's great to see.

You have people coming in all the time with the latest and greatest wines. What is the strangest sales pitch you've heard?

Gordy: I've had people come in and try to sell me their wine using just a Powerpoint presentation. When I asked them to see the wine, they don't have any but they still want to know if I'm interested. I say 'sure, but at least come back with some wine so I can taste it (laughing).' I've had people show up with no labels on the bottle or I'll ask how many bottles can they produce and they'll say maybe 10 per day. It's a shock to their system when I have to tell 'em I've got 1400 licencees to supply. There's never a lack of creativity out there.

How has your palate evolved?

Gordy: I think over the years it has gotten better (laughing), if that makes sense. I'll admit I can be tricked – on the good side and bad. However, I have several 'go to' people who I rely on. We also have tastings with our sales team and rate the wines or go to outsiders like Gar Winslow of Midland or Jeff Opperman of Saginaw for their opinions. We stretch WAY beyond my palate to be sure the wine is right for us. I'm old school – I still like Zinfindel, which was very popular 20 years ago and I'm really starting to like the new red blends that are coming out.

So, pick a wine that best describes you...

Gordy: It would be aged well, smooth, well balanced with a clean finish. I would pick Baron Rothschild...now I'm a bit embarrassed because I don't usually talk much about myself.

Ok, so let's make you the Czar of the wine distribution system...what would you change?

Gordy: (laughing) I knew you'd eventually get around to a loaded question. I'll just say we take great pride in adhering to all the regulations in the current system and we try very hard to please everyone involved.

With the growth of Fabiano Brothers over the last 125 years, I'd say their Wine Division is pleasing quite a few wine drinkers these days. Thanks Gordy.

My head says go to the gym.
My heart say drink more wine.

RETAILERS

THE BREW KREW IN TAWAS
Fine Wine, Food And Fun

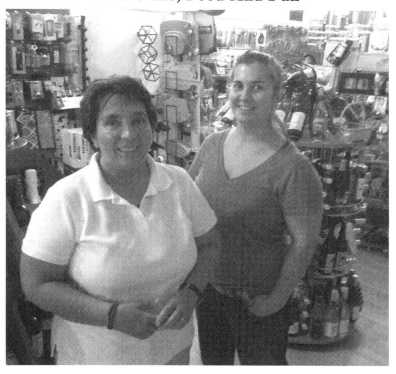

As you walk into the store, don't be surprised if you're asked 'hey, could you keep an eye on that child while I take care of a customer and then I'll be right with you.' The Brewer clan drafts you into the family and immediately makes you feel at home. And by the way, they also offer one of the best selections of Michigan wines on the sunrise side of the state.

Matriarch Diane Brewer saw a need in the community of Tawas and started the store in 1992 to fill a niche. "I wanted to create a retail experience that had a fun-family atmosphere and was a fun place to shop," she said. "We started with bath and kitchen accessories, then added gourmet foods and then wines."

It takes only one trip to the store to realize the name Brew Krew really fits but initially...

Diane said, "A marketing 'expert' talked me into using a K for Krew – all it did was confuse people at first but it makes us unique (laughing)."

Daughter Rebecca Buchanan came onboard to manage the food & wine side of the business and provide grandchildren to temporarily baby-sit. "It's hard to sell a product you're not personally committed to," she said. "I like products that I believe in and can stand behind – Michigan wines make that easy."

Interview with Diane Brewer and Rebecca Buchanan at Brew Krew:

You have such a great variety of Michigan wines. Is it difficult to pick one when advising a customer?

Rebecca: We can narrow it down by asking several things: if they have a palate preference: their price range and specifically what they want the wine for - that is before, during and after dinner. Their background or history with wine is also important before we make a recommendation

The store has evolved over time. Have you seen the wine drinkers evolve as well?

Rebecca: When we first made wines available the most recent boom in Michigan wineries was just beginning. Customers would look at anything but Michigan wines. Then gradually we noticed more and more people asking specifically for Michigan. I think in the beginning it was a 'let's support Michigan' attitude - now I think the majority of customers realize the quality of Michigan wines has improved and also warrants their attention. Our Michigan wine display continues to grow each year.

What type of wines are your biggest sellers?

Diane: Initially it was the sweeter wines but in the last few years we've seen an appreciation for all varieties. The sweet fruity wines still sell well but more people are specifically asking for dryer wines - whites and reds.

When you added wines to the store what resources did you used to get started?

Rebecca: Gar Winslow at Eastman Party Store in Midland was a great help in building our wine list. I did waitressing and bartending in college but didn't have the wholesale experience. I also relied on the sales reps. The bigger wineries have a good sales staff out there and the smaller ones are very passionate about their wines. They should be – they have good wines.

Has your personal palate influenced which wines are available here?

Rebecca: The accurate answer is yes and no (laughing). I like wine but have a diverse palate so I've always used a shotgun approach to drinking it. Yes, I have favorites but I've never shied away from trying new wines. That's good advice to a new wine drinker - you'll naturally want to gravitate to your favorites but always look to expand that list by experimenting.

You're always trying to educate the customer, right?

Diane: We have two wine tastings a year for that specific purpose. There are at least 40 different wines there and it helps educate us as well.

As a retailer, customer service is obviously paramount but the customer isn't always right - are you confronted with that problem with their wine requests?

Rebecca: The most frustrating thing we encounter is when a customer says 'I had this wine up north in a tasting room can you get that wine for me.' We are somewhat limited and dependent on distributors and if we aren't serviced by that particular wine distributor it's difficult to fill our customers need. It's also not very practical for us to drive to the winery and get it for them most of the time.

But isn't wine meant to take away the frustration?

Diane: We want to make the customers happier going out the door then when they came in. If they've got some wine with them it's probably a good start (laughing).

Meeting the Brew Krew is a good start to making anyone feel better. Thanks to the whole crew.
  See the Brew Krew ad on the back cover.

THE ROADS ALL LEAD TO DUSTY'S FOR WINE IN THE LANSING AREA

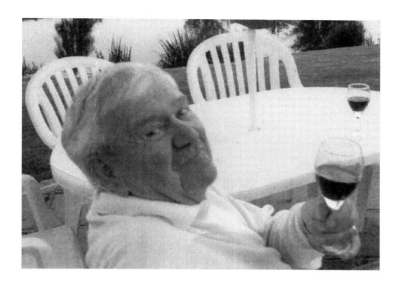

Dusty Rhodes was a visionary. He saw a need and tried to fill it. In some cases, he was way ahead of his time. But his business, Dusty's Cellar, has survived the test of time.

After spending time working in London, England and becoming acquainted with European style breads and wine, in 1980 Dusty opened a bakery on Grand River Ave. in Okemos. The next year, he built a wine shop with specialty foods called Dusty's Cellar. At that time, the surrounding land was primarily residential and agricultural.

Today, the business includes Dusty's Wine Bar (1986), Dusty's Tap Room (2004), four separate private meeting/dining areas added over the years and literally sits in the heart of a mega-commercial sprawl. When sipping a glass of wine on the patio at Dusty's, its hard to visualize a residential area across the street.

Dusty's son, Matt, started at the bottom of the employment chain, doing dishes and stocking the shelves. Now, he manages 80 employees and has continued Dusty's tradition of providing excellent customer service and sound advice when it comes to the perfect wine selection.

Interview with Matt Rhodes:

Dusty's Cellar carries a huge wine selection. How many are Michigan wines?

Matt: I haven't done the numbers recently but I would estimate we carry up to 1000 selections and around 100 are Michigan labels. The quality of in-state wines has increased dramatically. Ten years ago, Michigan wines took up a corner of the Cellar. Now, they would cover an entire wall.

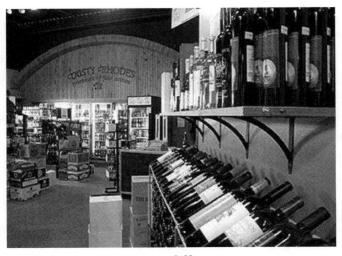

Are you noticing any trends with wine drinkers?

Matt: Twenty years ago, we sold a lot of white zinfandel but these days, just a fraction of those amounts. Now, as those wine drinkers get older, their palates tend to gravitate to a drier wine. With the younger wine drinker, Moscato D'Asti is selling off the charts – the new white zin.

When a new wine drinker asks for advice, what do you tell them?

Matt: Try to clear your mind of preconceived notions about what you think wine is supposed to taste like. Dry Rosé is a perfect example – they see Rosé and think sweet. But when it's chilled, they might think it was a white wine or if it were served at room temperature, they would say it was a red. Even we have to guard against our own prejudices – if I saw a Stag's Leap Cabernet, my expectations would be higher in comparison to a new California wine I wasn't familiar with. In Michigan, there are wineries starting up in non-traditional grape-growing areas, so we have to set aside those prejudices when trying their wines.

Dusty's has a great reputation for being the place to get good wine advice. How did you build up that reputation?

Matt: Certainly, my dad started that process. He was very knowledgeable and well liked. But Dusty's became more than a retail outlet. We have two sommeliers and a great chef on staff who are willing to assist our customers in pairing the right wine with the right occasion. Getting to know your customer base is a priority as well. Our Wine Bar General Manager is a huge supporter of in-state wines and is currently serving several Michigan wines by the glass.

The Wine Bar opened in 1986, yet "wine bars" are a fairly recently phenomenon. Dusty truly was a pioneer.

Matt: Yeah, it was called that from the day it opened and it's been a very successful addition to the Cellar. Ironically, when my dad opened the bakery in 1980, out in the "boondocks" everyone thought he was nuts. He installed a huge espresso & cappuccino machine – couldn't give the stuff away (laughing), no one knew what a latte was. Now, there's a coffee shop practically on every corner.

The Michigan wine industry is rife with "characters." It sounds like your dad qualified. Can you think of others?

Matt: Well, my dad certainly had a great reputation – in a good way – for being a character. Everybody loved to come in and see Dusty. He and Ed O'Keefe, of Chateau Grand Traverse, were great pals. It was a titanic battle to see who was the bigger BSer. I'd say it was a toss-up (laughing).

This is much more than a quaint little wine operation. What part of your job gives you the most satisfaction?

Matt: I get a sense of pride and satisfaction when I hear people say 'we depend on you.' Of course, we're not the only place in town but we have been around for a long time and have worked hard on customer service. So, I think it would really be a loss to the community if we weren't here.

What's on the horizon for Dusty's?

Matt: With the private dining areas – the Bordeaux Room, the Tuscan Room & the Leelanau Patio, we're scheduling larger meetings and gathering. We're putting on more special wine & food tasting events. For the purpose of educating our customers and entertainment, we're looking into coordinating a bus tour of Michigan wineries. We've always had a great relationship with the wineries and I think it would also be a lot of fun.

I would agree with that – sign me up! Thanks, Matt

I don't need an app that tells me how many calories I've burned. I need an app that tells me how many glasses of wine I've earned!

.

FOR GOOD WINE & GOOD WINE ADVICE IN MIDLAND GO TO EASTMAN PARTY STORE & GAR WINSLOW

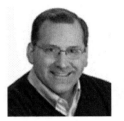

It seems every retail outlet has a liquor license these days – Target, Dollar General, Walgreens, gas stations, convenience stores...But where do you go to get good wine and good advice about wine? In Midland, it's Eastman Party Store and the wine expert is Gar Winslow.

Back in the days when the numbers of Michigan wineries were in the single digits and most wines had a twist off cap, costing fewer than five dollars, Eastman Party Store was one of the few places to get a bottle of wine with a cork and a good wine selection.

"It's hard to believe our store has been around for a half century," said current owner Gar Winslow. "The longevity is a tribute to good service." Built in the early 1960's by the Rapanos family, Ted Rezimer took over in 1970 after realizing Midland's desire to expand along Eastman Rd., which is the primary northern corridor.

Winslow grew up in Midland and remembers when the store was the only retail business on Eastman Rd. north of Saginaw Rd., which is the main east/west street. "When I was a kid, just two miles up from the store was all farm land. Today, there is the entire Mall complex and multiple hotels and restaurants there," he said. "I started working for Ted as a senior in high school and began working here full-time after getting a business degree from Northwood University."

"Ted was a family friend and he always told me if I was ever interested in becoming the owner, the store would be available for purchase, which I did in 1998."

After a series of expansions and renovations, Eastman Party Store has a highly respected wine list and Gar has developed a reputation for being 'spot on' in recommending the right wine for any occasion.

Interview with Gar Winslow:

What percentage of your business is wine, Michigan wine and how many employees to you have?

Gar: We have nine to 12 full and part-time employees. Roughly 27 % of the business is wine with 5% of that being Michigan wines.

Have you observed any changes in Michigan wines over the years?

Gar: People still think of Michigan wines as being sweet and fruity, not necessarily food wines. Many of the European vinifera – Chardonnay, Cabernet Franc, Pinot Noir are all starting to come into their own here in Michigan. If people will try them, they would realize those wines are very good as well.

Is there a trend of people going to drier wines here?

Gar: The fact is, here in Michigan, sweet still sells. I think most wineries would like to produce a drier wine but the cases of sweeter wines are the ones still moving the fastest out of the tasting rooms and the retailers are also seeing that. People with a more educated palate prefer dry but there are a lot of people who say they like dry but buy sweet (laughing). There is also a big push in the market for a sweet red – they are hearing from their doctors that it's good for you.

What advice would you give a novice wine drinker?

Gar: If it's a new customer or someone new to drinking wine, generally, I'd suggest a sweet wine to start. But I also suggest trying, say four different types of wine to begin with. Even if you find one that you like, don't stop searching because your taste does evolve. Keep 'advancing' your palate – it does change, even with the same wine. Many times people just stop looking after they find THE one, but if they do they are missing out on so many other great wines.

I'm sure you've heard a variety of 'unusual' questions from retail customers – any come to mind?

Gar: Well, it's hard to keep a straight face when you ask a customer if they prefer a dry wine and they say they would rather have a wet wine…especially when you realize they are being serious.

What questions should a customer ask that would help you suggest the right wine?

Gar: For us to make a good suggestion the critical information to start with is their price range, the types of wine they like and the occasion or food pairing. From there, we can narrow it down to a few wines that may meet their needs.

Are you dictated by regulation on wine pricing?

Gar: We are regulated on liquor but not for beer and wine. The only restriction on wine pricing is it has to be above cost. So the mark up is based on what we feel will cover our end costs. Most wineries don't make suggestions on pricing but we try to stay at or below their tasting room price.

From a retailer's standpoint, is closure an issue?

Gar: I prefer a cork – the industry has made great strides to eliminate a lot of the taint problems. I've found synthetic corked wines tend to oxidize much faster in many cases. But I have no problem with twist off caps, which I think has come on strong because of the cork problems in the past. We are compensated for cork problems from the distributors and wineries. Legally, we aren't required to compensate customers or maybe 'allowed' to compensate them but we do – common sense – you want to keep customers happy.

What sources do you use to educate yourself on what's available in Michigan wines?

Gar: I do read wine periodicals/magazines but now I mostly rely on my own palate through wine tastings with reps. When I was younger I read more books, which I would recommend to get an overall view of wines in general. But once you have the basics, it's all about taste.

Retail is a tough business. Do you still find your job satisfying?

Gar: It is tough and getting tougher all the time...but every time you see a repeat customer come through the door with a smile and a thank you for that 'last bottle of wine you recommended' or a new customer says they're here because of a recommendation from a regular customer – that keeps the doors open and makes me want to discover the next great wine.

We all appreciate that...thanks Gar.

The secret to enjoying a good wine: open the bottle to allow it to breathe and if it doesn't look like it's breathing, give it mouth to mouth.

IDEAL PARTY STORE IN BAY CITY
The Ideal Place To Go For Wines

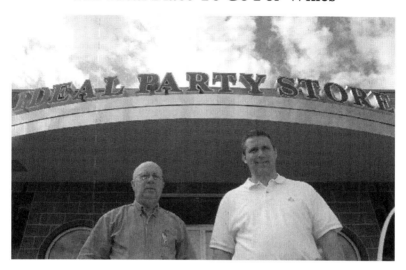

Jerry Crete's grandfather was visiting relatives down in East Detroit in May 1934. Prohibition had just ended and he noticed a few new stores had cropped up – they were called "party stores."

He had a bread route; times were tough but this was something he thought might catch on in Bay City – boy, did it ever. After scraping together the mattress money, the grocery money and a private stash buried in a can out back, a new business appeared on Johnson Street on the east side of Bay City called Ideal Beer Service Store.

At the time, there were three local breweries in Bay City and they made two or three deliveries daily to keep up with demand. Wine was eventually added and they sold a lot of champagne.

Most of it probably ended up in the Saginaw River due to celebrations for every launching from the Defoe Shipyard.

Jerry's father took over in the late 50's and liquor was added in 1962, which prompted a name change to Ideal Party Store.

Like father, like son – Jerry practically grew up in the store doing odd jobs for pop and candy, eventually drawing his first official paycheck in June 1979. He had to stick to dusting shelves and stocking because he was only fourteen and had to wait four more years to sell alcohol – by then he was managing the store.

After a college education in finance and several years in banking, the family business pulled him back when an opportunity came up to expand into Saginaw. He spent years building up business for both stores but the pull to be close to his family prompted selling the Saginaw store. Customers kept up the call 'when are you gonna open a store on the west side?' and in 2008 he did just that.

Now, with two stores in Bay City and over 1000 wine selections from $5 to $500, Jerry is the "wine guy" you go to for advice.

Interview with Jerry Crete:

How does wine get to your stores?

Jerry: Wine has always been delivered through a network of distribution companies. There used to be quite a few distributors but over the years they've been bought out by others. Now we deal with several very large ones and a few smaller companies.

The 3-tier system; winery to distributor to retailer has been in place for a long time. There's a push to eliminate the middle tier but I don't think it will happen.

Would that help or hurt the wine industry?

Jerry: In my opinion, it would hurt, especially the small wineries. Ironically, those seem to be the ones pushing to become their own independent distributor. For the most part, the current system works okay – be careful what you wish for.

Has there ever been a 'go-to' Michigan wine for you?

Jerry: One that comes to mind is Chateau Grand Traverse Late Harvest Riesling, which has been their flagship wine for years. When we had the money, I would order 50 cases in September. By mid-October, everybody was scrambling and by Thanksgiving, we'd be the only ones with a supply left. People would come in and buy it by the caseload – by Christmas, we'd be out too. But they make a lot more now and are in a lot more stores these days.

There is a price difference usually between the tasting rooms and the retail store. Why is that?

Jerry: Originally, it was cheaper to buy it in the tasting rooms. Through discussions between the wineries, distributors and retailers, we began to see a pricing change about 10 years ago. Wineries realized the need to be on par with retailers or even a bit higher to facilitate sales Monday through Friday. Customers weren't going to come to visit wineries every weekend to save a few bucks on the bottle price but if they were there, they would buy the wine anyway. Everyone benefited in the long run.

What percentage of your business is wine and what percent is Michigan wine?

Jerry: One third of the business is wine and nearly one third of that is Michigan wine. That percentage is increasing all the time as more wineries open in Michigan.

What advice would you give to people about wines?

Jerry: In general, people have a preconceived notion about what wine goes with certain foods. But I tell them not to drink a wine they don't like just because they think it's the proper one but also don't be afraid to try something new.

Have you noticed any trends in Michigan wines?

Jerry: First, the selection and quality is growing and getting better. They are hearing about the health benefits of red wines but still have the palate for sweet. So wines like Leelanau Cellars Sweet Red and Grand Traverse Sweet Red and Peninsula Cellars Detention are leaping off the shelf. Muscatos seem to be the popular wine today. More and more people want to support in-state wineries. More wines are coming out but I also think more people are drinking wine – even diehard beer drinkers are having a glass of wine with dinner.

Are you seeing more baby boomer customers or younger generation wine drinkers or is it remaining about the same?

Jerry: Starting about 20 years ago, I'm seeing people drink less alcohol in general. The drinking laws have something to do with that but also people aren't having 2 martini lunches or having a drink after work as much either. In the case of wine, they aren't buying 3 bottles of Boones Farm but rather a nice $12 bottle to go with dinner or share with friends – not much difference in money spent but going for higher quality.

So describe yourself by a Michigan wine...

Jerry: I'm a Chateau Fontaine Big Red Paw. That winery does a good job with all their wines but especially the reds. I'm a pushover for a good Michigan red.

I'll drink to that. Thanks Jerry.

You + me + a bottle of wine = Happiness!

WINE CLUBS IN MICHIGAN

Tasters Guild International – Grand Rapids Headquarters

There are 25 chapters around the country, with each chapter remaining somewhat autonomous. Michigan has eight chapters : Ann Arbor, Grand Rapids, Grand Traverse, Kalamazoo, Lake Shore (Grand Haven/Holland), Lapeer, Marshall and Oakland.

Annual membership is $45, which includes the Tasters Guild Journal published twice a year. Each chapter sponsors individual wine tastings and food/wine pairings. The organization sponsors the International Wine Judging contest in Grand Rapids every April and a Consumer's Wine Judging in April for members.

They sponsor two annual trips – a winter wine cruise and a summer outing to visit Europe's wine country. Visit their website and you can join online at, www.tastersguild.com.

From Tasters Guild President Joe Borrello: "Tasters Guild is not just for connoisseurs. It is intended to be a broad-based organization able to benefit all levels of consumers, from the novice to the professional."

Ann Arbor Chapter & The Ann Arbor Wine Club

President, Dick Scheer – The Village Corner

The Ann Arbor Wine Club started in 1973 and was originally called the Ann Arbor Wine & Food Society. The annual fee is $9 by email or $12 by postal mail and the Tasters Guild membership is $45 or $85 for two years. There are currently over 700 members between the two wine clubs. The Ann Arbor Club has six meetings annually and the Tasters Guild schedules twelve. There is a dinner/tasting scheduled every three weeks. Contact information is winestaff@villagecorner.com or visit the http://villagecorner.com website.

Grand Rapids Tasters Guild Chapter

The club started in 1974 and became a Tasters Guild chapter in 1987. There are 10-12 meeting per year with over 350 members. Contact Joe Borrello at joeb@tastersguild.com.

Kalamazoo Tasters Guild Chapter

The Kalamazoo Chapter was one of the original Tasters Guild groups. There are 9-11 meetings scheduled at area restaurants for food & wine pairing. They are registered as a non-profit educational organization ($45 annual fee) with 200 members. Charlotte Horton-Davis is the 2013 president. Contact information is tastersguildkzoo@aol.com.

Greater Lansing Vintners Club

The club started back in 1968 and currently has approx. 800 members. Twelve wine events are scheduled annually. Membership is $20/yr., $36/2 yrs., $50/3 yrs., senior (65+)/$18 and student/$15 per year, which includes an E-newsletter called *Wineline*. Mike Brenton is the current president. Contact information is glvintnersclub@gmailcom or visit the club website, www.glvintnersclub.com.

Bay City Wine Club

The club started in 2011 and currently has 272 members. They meet twelve times a year on the 3rd Wednesday of every month. Membership fee is one bottle of wine per person, a glass to sample and a hors d'oeuvre to pass. Jean Ann DeShano is the president. You can find contact information at the Bay City Wine Club on Facebook.

As this happens to be my 'home' wine club, I offer proof we have a great time!

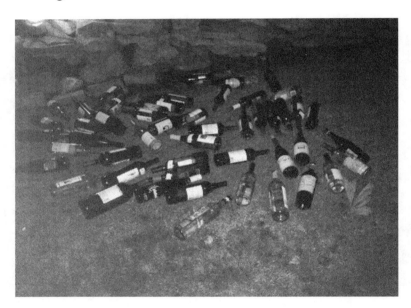

Other clubs:

American Wine Society
Detroit Chapter
Ed Nelson, Chair
www.americanwinesociety-michigan.com

Oakland Tasters Guild Chapter
Larry & Donna Palizza
lvpmgt@aol.com

Gibbs' Wine Tasters
$40 annual fee – nine events annually
Detroit East Side – Larry Shade
www.gibbswineshop.com

Cereal City Corkscrew Club
Mark Reincke, Battle Creek

Winetasters
Dennis or Dan Walsh, Rochester Hills

BIBLIOGRAPHY

American Cellars, *Wine Lover's Handbook*, 2011

Hathaway, Lorri & Kerrerreis, Sharon. *The History of Michigan Wines*. South Carolina: The History Press. 2010

Herbst, Lon & Sharon. *Wine Lover's Companion*, 2nd edition. New York: Barron's 2003

May, Danny. *The Only Wine Book You'll Ever Need*. Massachusetts: Adams Media 2004

Michigan Grape & Wine Industry Council. *Wine Country Magazine* 2010-2013

Ritz, Rebecca. "Women Prefer Wine With a Story To Tell." Jan. 19, 2013

Sood, Suemedha. "Travelwise: Answers from a Sommelier." *Food and Drink*. May 18, 2012

PHOTO CREDITS (photo source, page #)

Alpena News: 162; Appellation-America.com Eleanor/Ray Heald: 101, 196; Bay City Wine Club: 378; Bob Gudas: cover; Brandy Wheeler Traverse Traveler: 140,144; Chris Zimmerman: 347; Family Collections: 95,96(1-2), 106, 124, 260, 261, 267, 294, 315, 361; Jackson Citizen Patriot Dave Weatherwax: 310; Mari Kane: 278; Marshal King: 182; Michiganwine.com: 29, 91, 201; Mike Glinishi: 290, Mlive: 371; Ned Ewing: 63, 68; Ray Gudas: 220; Rick Sigsby: 70, 119, 184, 189, 192, 248, 304, 343, 351, 357; Trip Advisor: 156; Wine Dog USA: 301; Winery website/Facebook page: 21, 27, 32, 33, 38, 39, 41, 45, 47, 48, 50, 54, 56, 58, 78, 84, 87, 89, 111, 112, 114, 115, 126, 129, 134, 146, 167, 172, 177, 202, 208, 212, 215, 217, 223, 226, 231, 236, 242, 254, 273, 276, 280, 285, 299, 320, 324, 329, 330, 331, 333, 362, 366.

ABOUT THE AUTHOR

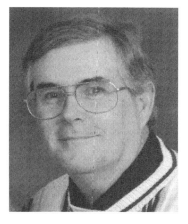

Rick Sigsby is a retired Park Ranger, writer and part-time owner of racehorses. He has a newspaper column called Rick Off The Record and is a regular contributor to several nationally circulated horse racing magazines.

A lifelong resident of Michigan, Rick lives with his wife Ann and cat Tommy in the mid-Michigan town of Coleman.

Other Books By Rick Sigsby:

Discovering Hidden Treasures Part I

Discovering Hidden Treasures Part II

Images of America: Gladwin County

The Valley of Athletes – Athletic Greats of the Saginaw Valley Conference from 1904-2009

LIVING ON THE EDGE – A History of Auto Racing In Michigan

For more information, to order additional copies, other books by Rick Sigsby or book signing dates visit: www.rsigsby.com

WINE DIRECTORY

Northeast

Dizzy Daisy Winery and Vineyard   989-269-2366
www.dizzydaisywinery.com

Modern Craft Winery   989-876-0270
www.moderncraftwinery.com

Nicholas's Black River   231-625-9060
www.nicholasblackriverwinery.com

Rose Valley Winery   989-685-9399
www.rosevalleywinery.net

Stoney Acres Winery   989-356-1041
www.stoneyacreswinery.net

Thunder Bay Winery   989-358-9463
www.thunderbaywinery.com

Valley Mist Vineyards   989-685-9096
www.valleymistvineyards.com

Northwest

Cadillac Winery   989-392-2044
www.cadillacwinery.com

Douglas Valley Organic Vineyards   231-887-3333
www.douglasvalley.net

Fox Barn Market and Winery   231-861-8150
www.foxbarnwinery.com

Harbor Springs   231-526-3276
www.harborspringswinery.com

Heavenly Vineyards   616-710-2751
http://heavenlyvineyards.weebly.com

Jomagrha Vineyards and Winery	231-869-4232 www.jomagrha.com
Krolczyk Cellars	231-464-5414 www.kcellars.com
Left Foot Charley	231-995-0500 www.leftfootcharley.com
Northern Natural Winery	231-943-1078 www.northernnaturalorganic.com
Oceana Winery & Vineyard	231-343-0038 www.oceanawinery.com
Pleasantview Vineyards	231-526-8100 www.pleasantviewwinery.us
Raftshol Vineyards	231-271-5650 www.raftsholvineyards.com
Royal Farms Winery	866-224-4801 www.royalfarmsinc.com
St. Ambrose Cellars	231-882-4456 www.stambrose-mead-wine.com

Northwest Leelanau

Bel Lago Vineyard & Winery	231-228-4800 www.bellago.com
Black Star Farms	231-994-1270 www.blackstarfarms.com
Blustone	231-256-0146 www.blustonevineyards.com
Boathouse Vineyards	231-256-7115 www.boathousevineyards.com
Boskydel Vineyard	231-256-7272 www.boskydel.com

Brengman Brothers Winery	231-946-2764 www.brengmanbrothers.com
Chateau de Leelanau	231-271-8888 www.chateaudeleelanau.com
Chateau Fontaine	231-256-0000 www.chateaufontaine.com
Cherry Republic Winery	800-206-6949 www.cherryrepublic.com
Ciccone Vineyard and Winery	231-271-5553 www.cicconevineyard.com
45 North Vineyard and Winery	231-271-1188 www.fortyfivenorth.com
French Valley	231-271-2675 www.corkyswinebar.com
Gill's Pier Vineyard and Winery	231-256-7003 www.gillspier.com
Good Harbor Vineyards	231-256-7165 www.goodharbor.com
Good Neighbor Organic	231-386-5636 www.goodneighbororganic.com
L. Mawby Vineyards	231-271-3522 www.lmawby.com
Laurentide Winery	231-994-2147 www.laurentidewinery.com
Leelanau Cellars	231-386-5201 www.leelanaucellars.com
Longview Winery LLC	231-228-2880 www.longviewwinery.com
Motovino	231-386-1027 www.motovinocellars.com

Shady Lane Cellars   231-947-8865
                                www.shadylanecellars.com

Silver Leaf Vineyard & Winery   231-271-3111
                                www.silverleafvineyard.com

Verterra Winery   231-256-2115
                                www.verterrawinery.com

Villa Mari Vineyards   231-256-2115
                                www.verterrawinery.com

Willow Vineyard   231-271-4810
                                www.willowvineyardwine.com

Northwest Old Mission

2 Lads Winery   231-271-3522
                                www.2LWinery.com

Black Star Farms - Old Mission 231-994-1300
                                ww.blackstarfarms.com

Bowers Harbor Vineyards   231-223-7615
                                www.bowersharbor.com

Brys Estate   231-223-9303
                                www.brysestate.com

Chateau Chantal Winery & Inn   800-969-4009
                                www.chateauchantal.com

Chateau Grand Traverse   231-223-7355
                                www.cgtwines.com

Hawthorne   231-929-4206
                                www.hawthornevineyards.com

Peninsula Cellars   231-933-9787
                                www.peninsulacellars.com

Southeast

Blue Water Winery and Vineyard	810-622-0328 www.bluewaterwinery.com
Burgdorf's Winery	517-655-2883 www.burgdorfwinery.com
Carriage House Cellars	810-632-7692 www.spicerswinery.com
Chateau Aeronautique Winery	517-569-2132 www.chateauaeronautiquewinery.com
Cherry Creek Cellars	517-531-3080 www.cherrycreekwine.com
Cherry Creek Old Schoolhouse	517-592-4663 www.cherrycreekwine.com
Fieldstone	248-656-0618 www.fieldstonewine.com
Flying Otter Winery	877-876-5580 www.flyingotter.com
Green Barn Winery	810-367-2400
Hometown	989-875-6010 www.hometowncellars.com
J. Trees Cellars	877-304-3254 www.treeswines.com
Lone Oak Vineyard Estate	517-522-8167 www.loneoakvineyards.com
Old Town Hall Winery	810-359-5012 www.oldtownhallwinery.com
Pentamere Winery	517-423-9000 www.pentamerewinery.com

Sandhill Crane Vineyards　　　　517-764-0679
　　　　　　　　　　　　　　　　www.sandhillcranevineyards.com

Sandy Shores Winery　　　　　　810-327-6394
　　　　　　　　　　　　　　　　www.mccallumorchard.com

Sleeping Bear Winery　　　　　　517-531-7777
　　　　　　　　　　　　　　　　www.sleepingbearwine.com

Uncle John's Fruit House Winery　989-224-3686
　　　　　　　　　　　　　　　　www.fruithousewinery.com

Village Winery　　　　　　　　　586-337-2563
　　　　　　　　　　　　　　　　www.villagewineryromeo.com

Wolcott Winery　　　　　　　　　810-789-9561
　　　　　　　　　　　　　　　　www.wolcottwinery.com

Southwest

12 Corners Vineyards　　　　　　269-637-1211
　　　　　　　　　　　　　　　　www.12corners.com

Cascade Winery　　　　　　　　　616-656-4665
　　　　　　　　　　　　　　　　www.cascadecellars.com

Clay Avenue Cellars　　　　　　　231-722-3108
　　　　　　　　　　　　　　　　www.clayavenuecellars.com

Cody Kresta Vineyards and Winery　269-668-3800
　　　　　　　　　　　　　　　　www.codykrestawinery.com

Contessa Wine Cellars　　　　　　269-468-5534
　　　　　　　　　　　　　　　　www.contessawinecellars.com

Country Mill Winery　　　　　　　517-543-1019
　　　　　　　　　　　　　　　　www.countrymill.com

Domaine Berrien Cellars　　　　　269-473-9463
　　　　　　　　　　　　　　　　www.domaineberrien.com

Fenn Valley Vineyards　　　　　　269-561-2396
　　　　　　　　　　　　　　　　www.fennvalley.com

Founders Wine Cellar	269-426-5222 www.founderswinecellar.com
Free Run Cellars	269-471-1737 www.freeruncellars.com
Gravity	269-471-9463 www.gravitywine.com
Hickory Creek Winery	269-422-1110 www.hickorycreekwinery.com
Karma Vista Vineyards	269-468-9463 www.karmavista.com
Lake Effect Winery	231-747-8079 www.lakeeffectwinery.com
Lawton Ridge Winery	269-372-9463 www.lawtonridgewinery.com
Lehman's Orchard	269-683-9078 www.lehmansorchard.com
Lemon Creek Winery	269-471-1321 www.lemoncreekwinery.com
McIntosh Apple Orchards	269-637-7922 www.mcintoshorchards.com
Old Shore Vineyards	269-422-1967 www.oldshorevineyards.com
Peterson & Sons Winery	269-629-9755 www.naturalwine.net
Robinette Cellars	800-400-8100 www.robinettes.com
Round Barn Winery,	800-716-9463 www.roundbarnwinery.com
St. Julian Winery	269-657-5568 www.stjulian.com

Tabor Hill	800-283-3363
	www.taborhill.com
Warner Vineyards	800-756-5357
	www.warnerwines.com
White Pine Winery and Vineyards	269-281-0098
	www.whitepinewinery.com
Wyncroft	by appt.
	www.wyncroftwine.com

Upper Peninsula

Garden Bay Winery	906-361-0318
	www.gardenbaywinery.com
Mackinaw Trail Winery	231-487-1910
	www.mackinawtrailwinery.com
Northern Sun Winery	906-399-9212
S U & D Winery	906-226-1122
Threefold Vine Winery	906-644-7089

THE WINE DIRECTORY SPONSORS

Dusty's Cellar..391
12 Corners...392
45 North..393
Baroda Founders...394
Blustone..395
Brys Estate..396
Burgdorfs..397
Cadillac...398
Chateau Chantal..399
Chateau Grand Traverse 400
Cody Kresta 401
Contessa Cellars..402
Fenn Valley..403
Fox Barn 404
Good Harbor..405
Green Barn 406
Hawthorne Vineyards 407
Heavenly Vineyards...408
Karma Vista 409
Mackinaw Trail...410
Northern Natural 411
Pentamere..412
Robinette's..413
Rose Valley...414
Sandy Shores...415
St. Julian...416
Uncle John's Fruit House Winery........................417
Eastman Party Store..418

Please take the time to thank these sponsors for their support of this book project.

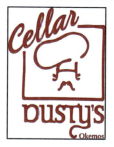

GREAT WINE
GREAT FOOD
GREAT FUN

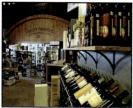

Dusty's Cellar - Retail for wine, beer, specialty foods, fresh pastries and more

Dusty's Wine Bar - fine dining in a relaxed bistro atmosphere

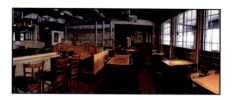

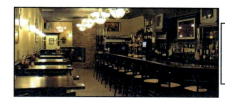

Dusty's Tap Room - your local neighborhood bar serving traditional pub fare, full bar and craft beer

© 2001-2013 Dusty's Cellar All Rights Reserved
Dusty's Cellar • 1839 Grand River Avenue • Okemos, Michigan 48864
Phone: 517.349.5150 • Fax: 517.349.8416
• Email: Dustys@Dustyscellar.com

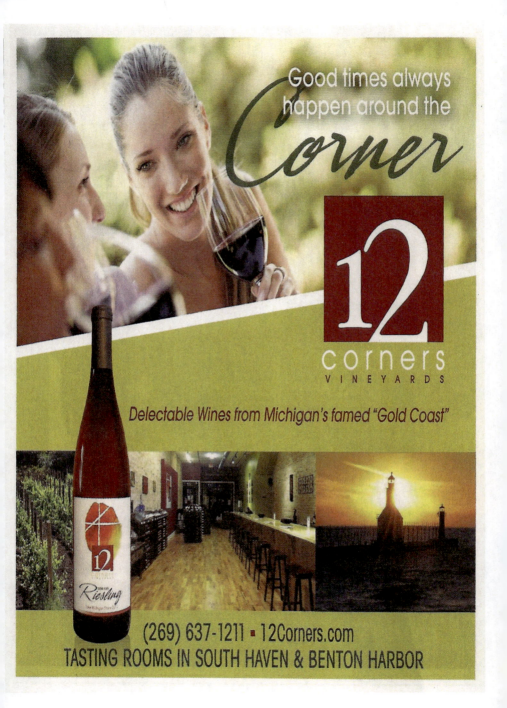

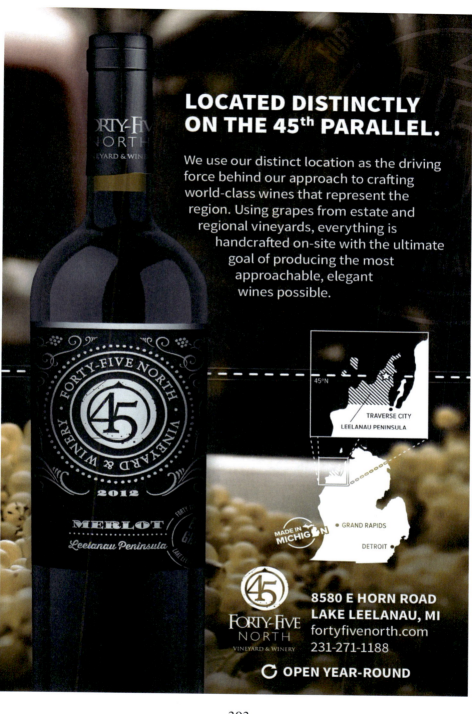

BARODA FOUNDERS
WINE CELLAR

Located at the corner of days-of-old charm and young-at-heart spirit. We enjoy sharing our wine, knowledge and good times!

Wine Tasting Room Hours
Sunday – Thursday 12pm-6pm
Friday – Saturday 12pm-8pm

8963 Hills Road ~ Baroda, Michigan 49101
Tel: 269-426-5222
www.founderswinecellar.com

NEW TASTING ROOM IN ST. JOSEPH
Sunday – Thursday 12pm- 8pm
Friday – Saturday 12pm-10pm
415 State St.

"Blustone is a hot new player on the Leelanau Peninsula." - *Traverse Magazine*

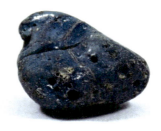

uniquely made.
undeniably leelanau.

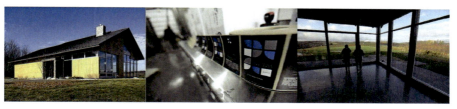

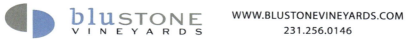

WWW.BLUSTONEVINEYARDS.COM
231.256.0146

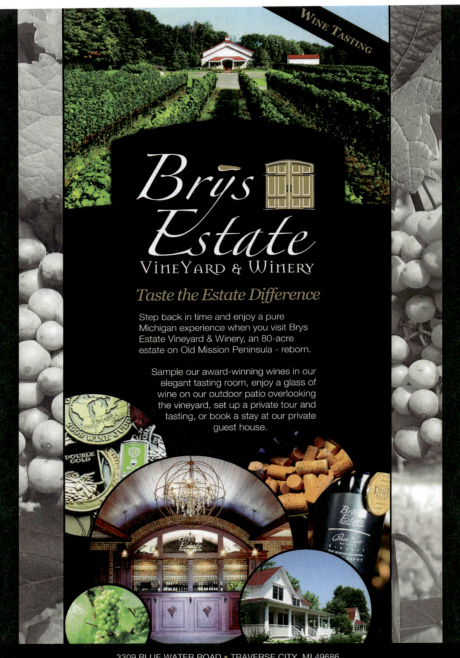

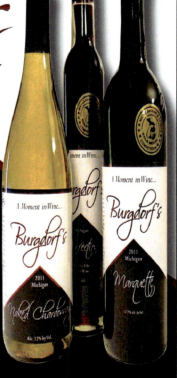

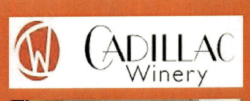
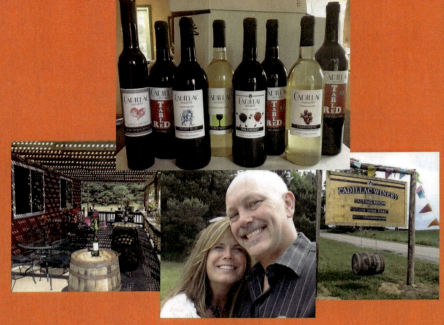

JOIN US
WHERE WINE LIVES

17480 18 MILE RD.
LEROY, MI. 49655
TAKE THE TUSTIN EXIT OFF US-131 EAST
JUST ELEVEN MILES SOUTH OF CADILLAC

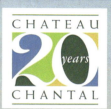

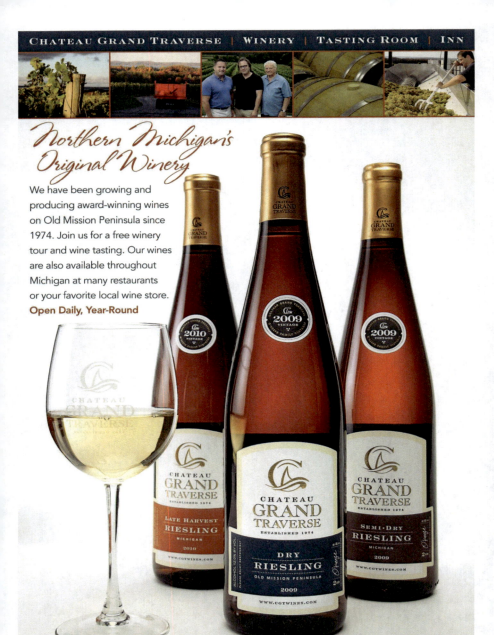

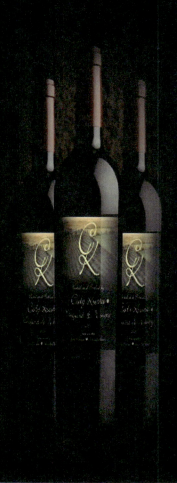

A place where quality wine is made
The place to go for a quality tasting experience

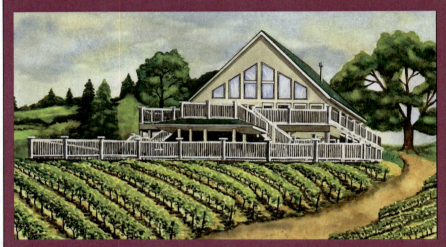

Life is there… you just have to taste it!

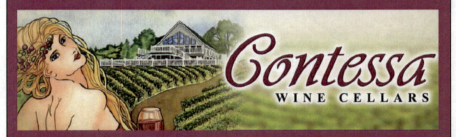

3235 Friday Rd.
Coloma, Michigan
269-468-5534

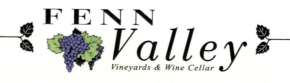

Enjoy a true **farm to bottle experience**.
Visit Fenn Valley Vineyards & Wine Cellar and sample from more than 25 award winning wines.

You'll discover what we mean when we say it's...
the lake effect everyone loves.

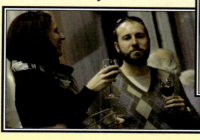

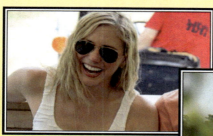

Free wine tasting
Wine tasting tours
Award winning wines
Winery direct discounts

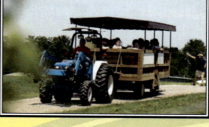

/fennvalley

6130 - 122nd Ave.
Fennville, MI 49408
I-196 exit 34, follow the "winery" signs.
Open year around. Check our website for hours
800-432-6265 www.fennvalley.com

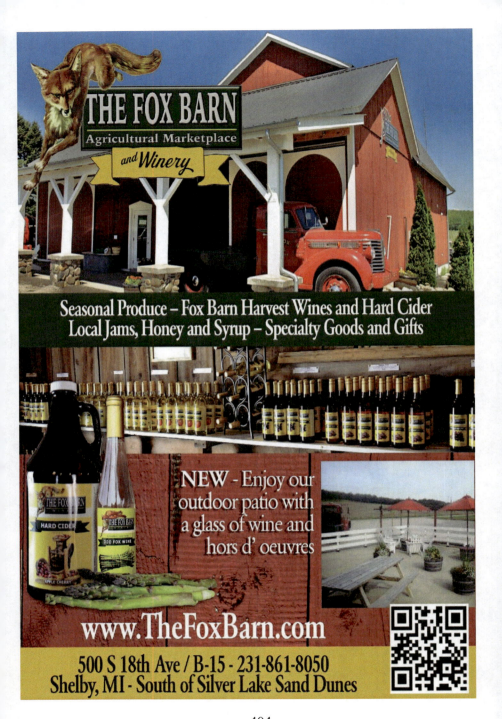

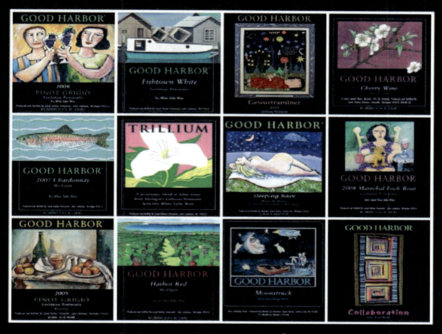

Green Barn

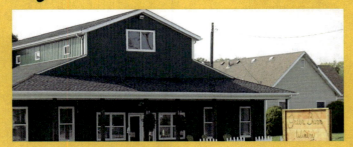

Winery

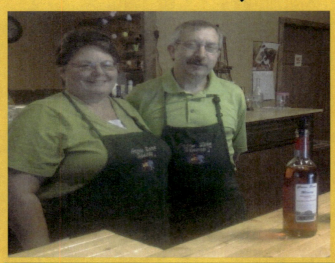

775 N. WADHAMS RD.
SMITHS CREEK, MI 48074
W-F 12-6 SAT.- 12-7 SUN.- 12-5

HAWTHORNE
VINEYARDS

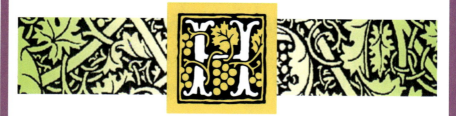

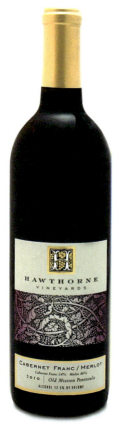

OLD MISSION PENINSULA'S
SECLUDED WEST BAY WINERY

From wine what sudden friendship springs!
John Gay 1738

OPEN MAY-OCT
OUTDOOR PATIO

BAYS VIEWS • AT APPROXIMATLY
9600 PENINSULA DR.

231-929-4206
HAWTHORNEVINEYARDS.COM
1000 CAMINO MARIA
TRAVERSE CITY, MI 49686

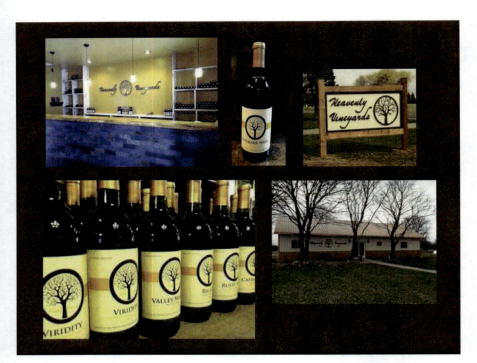

Heavenly Vineyards

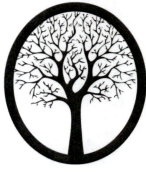

Wines Produced and Bottled In Morley, Michigan

15946 Jefferson road - Morley, MI

(616) 710-2751

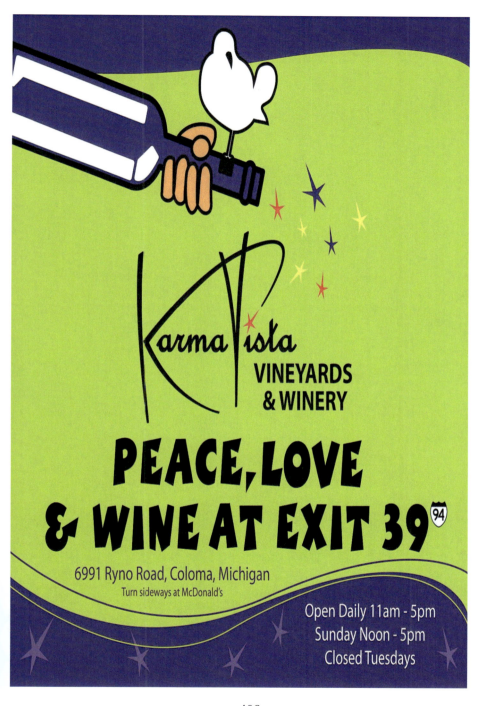

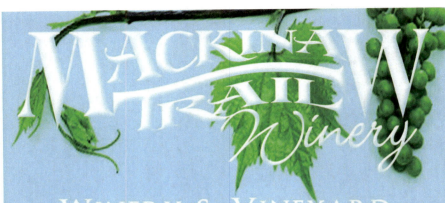

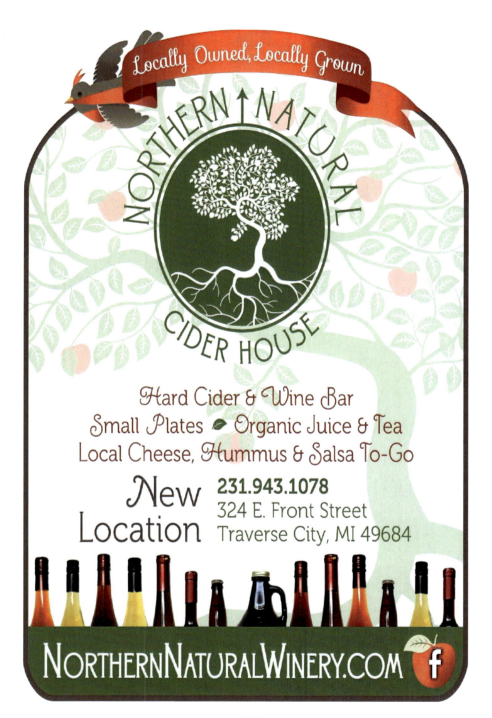

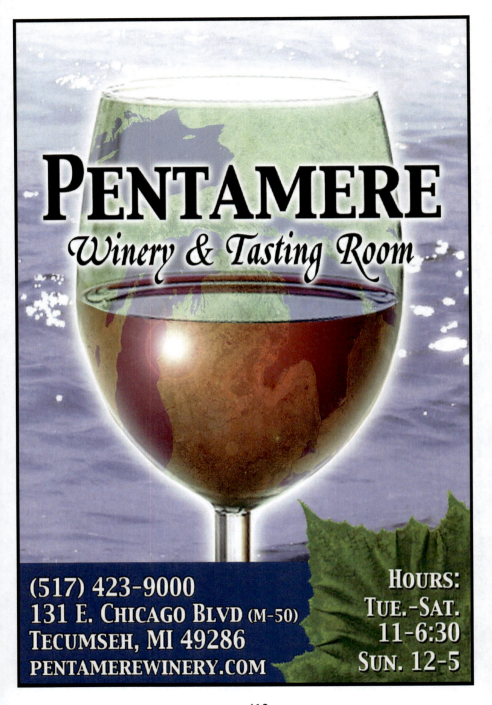

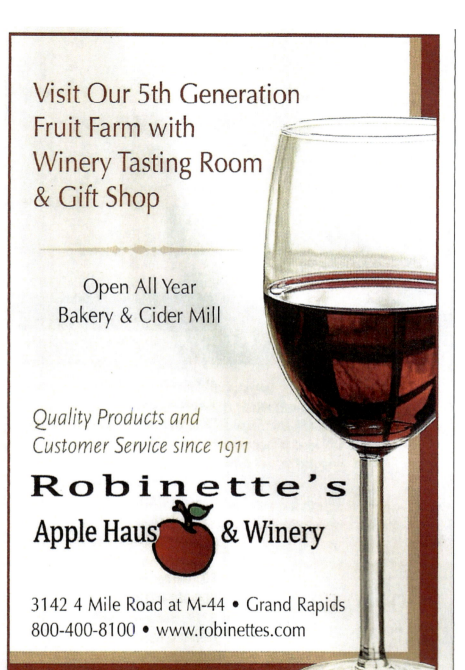

Live Well.
Love Much.
Laugh Often.

Hours:

Mon   11-5

Tues 11-5

Wed   Closed

Thur 11-5

Fri   11-5

Sat   11-5

Sun   12-4:30

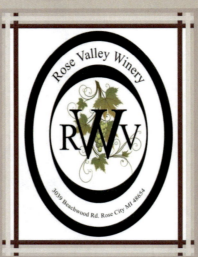

Free Tours

Free Tastings

Wine Gifts

Gift Certificates

Featuring Brownwood Farms

Rose Valley Winery

3039 Beechwood Rd.

Rose City, MI 48654

(989) 685-9399

Rosevalleywinery@m33access.com

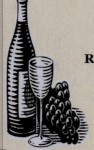

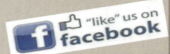

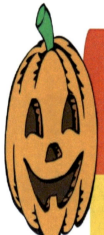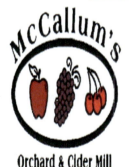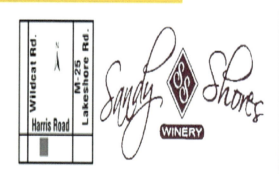

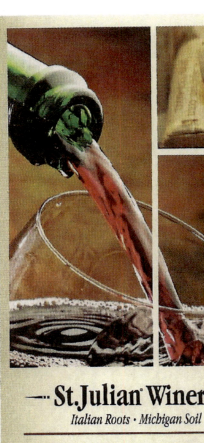
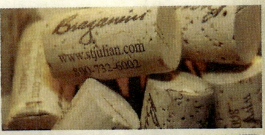
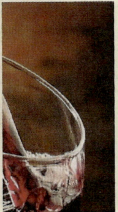
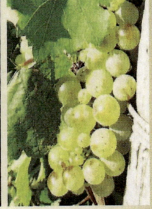
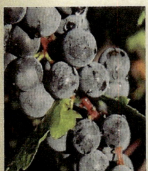
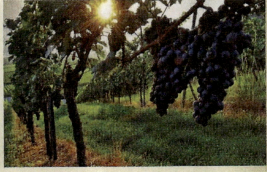

There are three reasons to try Uncle John's Hard Cider...

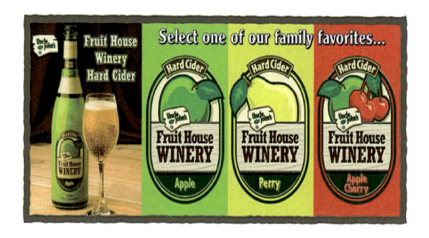

and fifty different reasons to visit
Uncle John's Cider Mill & Fruit House Winery.

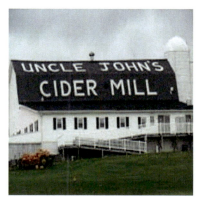
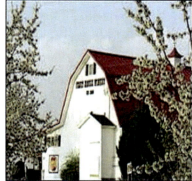

Read why you should on page 320.

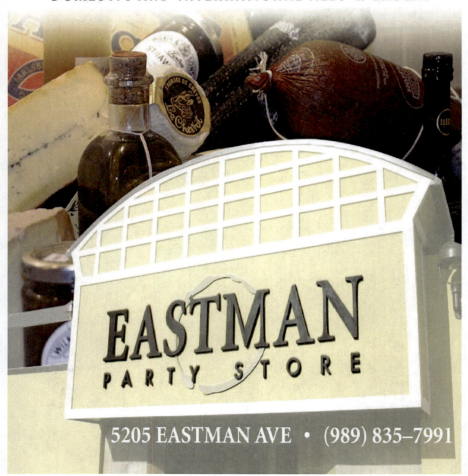